Assessing Human Exposure to Key Chemical Carcinogens

Vladan Radosavljevic

Assessing Human Exposure to Key Chemical Carcinogens

Diagnostic Approaches and Interpretation

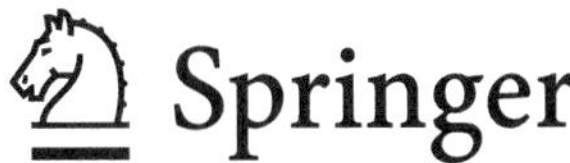

Vladan Radosavljevic
Military Medical Academy
Institute of Epidemiology
Crnotravska 17, 11000 Belgrade, Serbia

ISBN 978-3-031-84443-0   ISBN 978-3-031-84441-6   (eBook)
https://doi.org/10.1007/978-3-031-84441-6

This Springer imprint is published by the registered company Springer Nature Switzerland AG
The registered company address is: Gewerbestrasse 11, 6330 Cham, Switzerland

If disposing of this product, please recycle the paper.

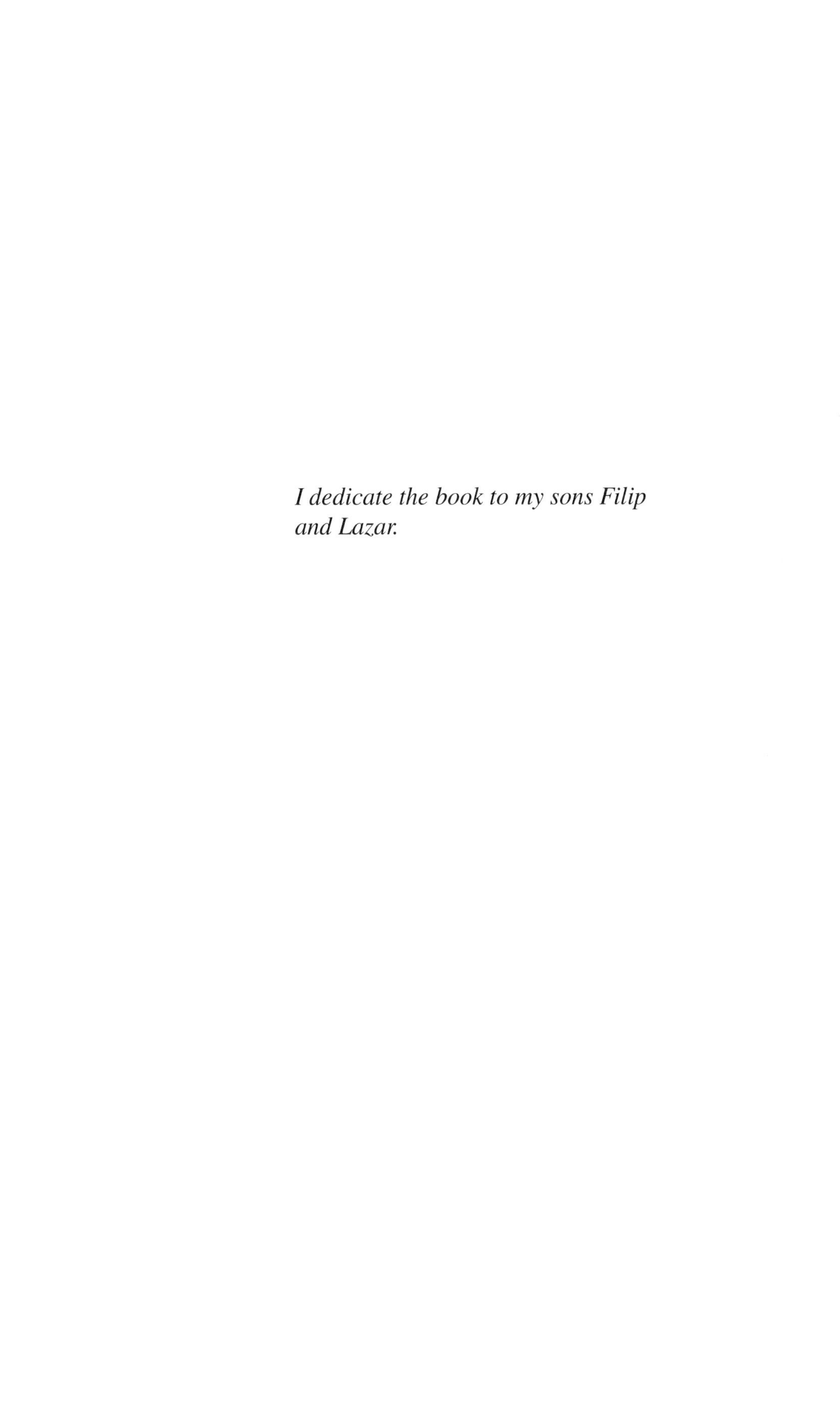

I dedicate the book to my sons Filip and Lazar.

Many data on the use of chemicals are still unknown, so we are unaware of many harmful exposures. It is not possible to eliminate carcinogens, but we could improve their detection and monitoring in the body (by special analyses of human urine) and thus define prevention measures that will lead to the reduction of their levels in the body. This is primarily the task of preventive oncology, ecology, and technology. Unfortunately, all the listed chemical carcinogens in this book have been used for decades, and some for centuries, without first examining their effects on human health. That mistake was paid for with millions of human lives. One must seriously think about the long-term effects of the products in use. Most of the carcinogens presented in the book have a cumulative effect.

By qualitative and quantitative determination of urinary markers of exposure to the most dangerous chemical carcinogens, it is possible to detect, eliminate, or reduce their sources, and with this strategy in a relatively short period, a significant step forward in preventive oncology could be made. This book focuses on chemical human carcinogens, i.e., group 1 carcinogens according to the International Agency for Research on Cancer. There are chemical carcinogens that break down into carbon dioxide and water and therefore have no measurable urinary metabolites (formaldehyde, acetaldehyde, ethyl alcohol, etc.).

This scientific volume provides theoretical and practical information on the diagnostics and interpretation of human contamination with the most important chemical carcinogens.

Preventive medicine, clinical medicine and other areas are systematically classified and focused on the primordial level of prevention. Special emphasis is put on finding sources of the most important chemical carcinogens and routes of human contamination.

Applications of approaches presented in the volume may reduce or eliminate human contamination with the most important chemical carcinogens and consequently the possibility of malignant disease occurrence as well as many other diseases (cardiovascular, endocrine, neurological, hematological, dermatological, etc.). The methodology presented in the volume is highly effective (comprising all the most important chemical carcinogens, with additional high sensitivity in their detection), affordable (based on the existing chemical devices and medical infrastructure), applicable (may be applied anywhere with HPLC and ICP devices), noninvasive (only a sample of urine is requested), quick (a dozen of minutes), and cheap (a couple of dozen Euros). The author hopes that the volume will serve for the development, improvement, and/or implementation of the screening method, preferably for malignant diseases.

The author is thankful to the Springer's editors Daniela Heller and Niveka Somasundaram for the time and effort invested to provide expert, insightful, and constructive suggestions that improved the chapters significantly.

Belgrade, Serbia   Vladan Radosavljevic
February, 2025

Contents

Introduction to the Screening of Urinary Biomarkers/Metabolites of the Key Chemical Carcinogens

1.1 Overview

Approximately, yearly and globally, almost 20 million people get sick and almost 10 million people die from all cancers. This book elaborates the chemical elements and chemical compounds that very probably contribute to both cancer occurrence in over 13.5 million people and death from cancer in over seven million people [1–4]. Moreover, chemical elements and chemical compounds very probably contribute to cancer occurrence in about 68% of all cancer cases and very probably significantly contribute to cancer death in about 72% of all cancer deaths (yearly and globally).

There are two main reasons for increasing cancer cases in the next decades: first, growing of the world population and, second, unproportional growing of the elderly population. Consequently, by 2050, the number of cancer cases is predicted to reach 35 million [5].

Classical malignancy screening detects people who already have malignancy and is often invasive and expensive. Here, the focus is on human chemical carcinogens (Group 1, according to IARC [International Agency for Research on Cancer] monographs, volumes 1–127) for which metabolites in urine are known. People could be tested for urinary metabolites according to different indications: hereditary factor, lifestyle, targeted studies, occupational exposure, environment, etc. The author hopes that this book will be a significant step forward in preventive oncology and an inspiration for further progress in the fight against malignant diseases [6].

1.2 Types of Carcinogens

According to the IARC classification, there are over 120 substances identified as very dangerous carcinogens (Group 1) [6]. The criteria for classification by groups are based on scientific data from the literature. In this book, we will focus on Group 1 human chemical carcinogens.

V. Radosavljevic, *Assessing Human Exposure to Key Chemical Carcinogens*, https://doi.org/10.1007/978-3-031-84441-6_1

Tobacco is a well-known carcinogen and is classified as a Group 1 carcinogen according to IARC (tobacco smoking, chewing tobacco, passive smoking—inhaling tobacco smoke from nearby smokers).

1.2.1 Chemical Carcinogens

Several Group 1 substances are antimalignant drugs currently used in clinical practice and are not discussed in this book (cyclosporine, busulfan, thiotepa, cyclophosphamide, chlornaphazine, azathioprine, etoposide in combination with cisplatin and bleomycin, etoposide, chlorambucil, treosulfan, methoxsalen/8-methoxylan, methoxylan, combination chemotherapy including alkylating agents, semustine). Furthermore, some carcinogens do not have specific metabolites in urine (urinary metabolites), but give water and carbon dioxide as final metabolites of the human body (acetaldehyde, formaldehyde, ethanol in alcoholic beverages). Strong inorganic acid mists (sulfuric and hydrochloric acid mists) do not have reliable final metabolites in the human body (metabolites in urine). Several hormonal drugs were excluded from further consideration (estrogen therapy, postmenopausal hormone therapy, combined estrogen-progestogen menopausal therapy, combined estrogen-progestogen oral contraceptives, diethylstilbestrol), as well as analgesic mixtures containing phenacetin (the cause of the so-called phenacetin kidneys), because they are well known as harmful substances or are under controlled use.

Some industrial processes have a carcinogenic effect, and due to the unclear and mixed effect of several compounds on the occurrence of malignancy, they were not taken into account in this review (production of isopropyl alcohol using a strong acid, production of aluminum, production of auramine, casting of iron and steel, production of magenta, production of rubber, welding fumes). Bis(chloromethyl) ether and chloromethyl methyl ether have rapid hydrolysis in the human body to hydrochloric acid and formaldehyde, without safe urinary metabolites. Aristolochic acids, aflatoxins, and some other carcinogens (to a much lesser extent) give DNA adducts that can be considered as a type of urinary carcinogen marker. However, their detection and interpretation of results requires additional research and processing. Nitrates, nitrites, and nitrosamines do not have specific urinary markers. The attempt to detect and indicate carcinogenic indicators in some foods, such as processed and red meat, is not complete (requires additional research and treatment in another book), and other much less important foods are not analyzed in the book (*Areca* nut).

Carcinogens listed as "outdoor air pollution," "soot" (exposure at the workplace of chimney sweeps), "painting" (exposure at the workplace), "indoor emissions from household combustion," "coke production," "gasification coal," "coal tar distillation," and "tar pitch" are quite broad and complicated to analyze. They could be analyzed through analyses of their carcinogenic components.

Carcinogenesis may last decades, and before malignant disease occurs, many other nonmalignant diseases/disorders appear caused or supported by chemical carcinogens (Table 1).

Table 1 Nonmalignant disorders/diseases caused by the most dangerous chemical carcinogens

Chemical carcinogens	Nonmalignant disorders/diseases	Sources
Inorganic arsenic	Dermatologic lesions and peripheral neuropathy	Prakash, PR; Narayan, A; Jain, S; Wig, N. Chronic arsenic poisoning: a sinister cause of peripheral neuropathy in a young couple. Journal of Postgraduate Medicine 70(2):p 105–108, Apr–Jun 2024. https://doi.org/10.4103/jpgm.jpgm_708_23
	Bronchitis, asthma	Kathryn Ramsey, 13—Arsenic and respiratory disease, Editor(s): Swaran Jeet Singh Flora, Handbook of arsenic toxicology (second edition), Academic Press, 2023, Pages 381–394, https://doi.org/10.1016/B978-0-323-89847-8.00013-4.
	Hepatic, endocrine, renal, neurological, hematological, immune, and cardiovascular disorders	Martínez-Castillo M, García-Montalvo EA, Arellano-Mendoza MG, et al. Arsenic exposure and non-carcinogenic health effects. Human & Experimental Toxicology. 2021;40(12_suppl):S826–S850. https://doi.org/10.1177/09603271211045955
	Pigmentation, depigmentation, and keratosis	Mazumder, D. N. G. (2007). Arsenic and non-malignant lung disease. *Journal of Environmental Science and Health, Part A*, *42*(12), 1859–1867. https://doi.org/10.1080/10934520701566926
	Hypertension, diabetes mellitus, cardiovascular diseases, and respiratory diseases	Chien-Jen Chen, Shu-Li Wang, Jeng-Min Chiou, Chin-Hsiao Tseng, Hung-Yi Chiou, Yu-Mei Hsueh, et al. Arsenic and diabetes and hypertension in human populations: A review, Toxicology and Applied Pharmacology, 222(3); 2007, 298–304. https://doi.org/10.1016/j.taap.2006.12.032 Katherine A. Moon, Eliseo Guallar, Jason G. Umans, et al. Association Between Exposure to Low to Moderate Arsenic Levels and Incident Cardiovascular Disease: A Prospective Cohort Study. Ann Intern Med.2013;159:649–659. [Epub 19 November 2013]. https://doi.org/10.7326/0003-4819-159-10-201311190-00719 Chen, Y., Parvez, F., Gamble, M., Islam, T., Ahmed, A., Argos, M., Graziano, J.H., & Ahsan, H. (2009). Arsenic exposure at low-to-moderate levels and skin lesions, arsenic metabolism, neurological functions, and biomarkers for respiratory and cardiovascular diseases: Review of recent findings from the Health Effects of Arsenic Longitudinal Study (HEALS) in Bangladesh. Toxicology and Applied Pharmacology, Available online 27 January 2009. https://doi.org/10.1016/j.taap.2009.01.010
	Arsenic-induced changes in the biomarkers reflecting oxidative stress, inflammation, dyslipidemia, vasoconstriction, monocyte adhesion, and angiogenesis, all related to promoting atherosclerosis and hypertension. Determinations of glucose intolerance, serum insulin and creatinine, and lean body mass suggested a potential role of arsenic-induced skeletal muscle atrophy and its association with insulin resistance. Respiratory function tests and measurements of serum immunoglobulin E and cytokines showed that arsenic-induced T helper 2 (Th2)-dominant immunomodulation might predispose to developing Th2-high-type asthma	Seiichiro Himeno, Khaled Hossain, Non-malignant diseases associated with environmental arsenic exposure in Taiwan, Chile, and Bangladesh, Metallomics Research, 2021, Volume 1, Issue 1, Pages rev-31–rev-46, Released on J-STAGE February 10, 2022

(continued)

Table 1 (continued)

Chemical carcinogens	Nonmalignant disorders/diseases	Sources
	Peripheral vascular diseases (black foot disease, a severe form of peripheral vascular disease, in which the blood vessels in the lower limbs are severely damaged, resulting eventually in progressive gangrene; Raynaud's syndrome, constriction of the small arteries in fingers and toes), skin lesions (dyspigmentation, keratoses), cardiovascular and cerebrovascular diseases, diabetes mellitus, neurological diseases, and diseases of the respiratory tract, the liver, and the spleen	Schuhmacher–Wolz, U., Dieter, H. H., Klein, D., & Schneider, K. (2009). Oral exposure to inorganic arsenic: evaluation of its carcinogenic and non-carcinogenic effects. *Critical Reviews in Toxicology*, *39*(4), 271–298. https://doi.org/10.1080/10408440802291505
Cadmium	Renal tubular dysfunction, cardiovascular diseases	Nishijo, M., Nakagawa, H. (2019). Effects of cadmium exposure on life prognosis. In: Himeno, S., Aoshima, K. (eds) Cadmium toxicity. Current topics in environmental health and preventive medicine. Springer, Singapore. https://doi.org/10.1007/978-981-13-3630-0_5
Nickel	*Nickel allergic contact dermatitis*	Samuel Buxton, Emily Garman, Katherine E. Heim, Tara Lyons-Darden, Christian E. Schlekat, Michael D. Taylor, Adriana R. Oller. Concise review of nickel human health toxicology and ecotoxicology. *Inorganics* 2019, *7*(7), 89; https://doi.org/10.3390/inorganics7070089
	The finding suggested that the occurrence of CHDs may be associated with nickel exposure	Zhang, Nannan PhDa; Chen, Ming MMb; Li, Jun MMc; Deng, Ying PhDa; Li, Sheng-li MDd; Guo, Yi-xiong MBAa; Li, Nana PhDa; Lin, Yuan MMe; Yu, Ping MDa; Liu, Zhen PhDa; Zhu, Jun MDa. Metal nickel exposure increase the risk of congenital heart defects occurrence in offspring: a case-control study in China. Medicine 98(18):p e15352, May 2019. https://doi.org/10.1097/MD.0000000000015352
	Allergy, cardiovascular and kidney diseases, lung fibrosis	Genchi, G.; Carocci, A.; Lauria, G.; Sinicropi, M.S.; Catalano, A. Nickel: human health and environmental toxicology. *Int. J. Environ. Res. Public Health* **2020**, *17*, 679. https://doi.org/10.3390/ijerph17030679
Beryllium	Chronic granulomatous lung disease, now termed chronic beryllium disease (CBD)	**Genetic and exposure risks for chronic beryllium disease.** Maier, Lisa A Clinics in Chest Medicine, Volume 23, Issue 4, 827–839
	Chronic beryllium disease	Infante, Peter F et al. Beryllium exposure and chronic beryllium disease. The Lancet, Volume 363, Issue 9407, 415–416.
Chromium VI	Occupational asthma (skin sensitizer) cause dermal irritation and ulceration, particularly on damaged skin, abnormal liver function, social memory loss, depression, schizophrenia, autism, olfactory dysfunction, polyneuropathy, chronic renal failure, and disrupted postimplantation development	Brandon M. Reif; Brian P. Murray. Chromium toxicity 2024, StatPearls Publishing LLC.

Aflatoxin	Weakened immune system	Abd Aziz Shamsudin, N., Oyebamiji, Y., ADEBAYO, I., Umar, O., Mohd Zaini, N., Ismail, M. Occurrence, health implications, and management of aflatoxin in cereal: a current review. *Egyptian Journal of Botany*, 2024; 64(4): 1–15. https://doi.org/10.21608/ejbo.2023.196133.2265; Monger, A., Mongar, P., Dorji, T. *et al.* The occurrence and human health risk assessment of total and aflatoxin B_1 in selected food commodities in Bhutan. *Sci Rep* **14**, 16258 (2024). https://doi.org/10.1038/s41598-024-63677-6
	Liver cirrhosis	Mirghani A. Yousif, CHAPTER 21—Aflatoxins in liver disease, Editor(s): Jose Debes, Treatment and management of tropical liver disease, Elsevier, 2025, Pages 176-181, ISBN 9780323870313, https://doi.org/10.1016/B978-0-323-87031-3.00030-5.
	Fetal growth abnormalities	Alameri MM, Kong AS, Aljaafari MN, Ali HA, Eid K, Sallagi MA, Cheng WH, Abushelaibi A, Lim SE, Loh JY, Lai KS. Aflatoxin contamination: an overview on health issues, detection and management strategies. Toxins (Basel). 2023 Mar 28;15(4):246. https://doi.org/10.3390/toxins15040246. PMID: 37104184; PMCID: PMC10140874.
Benzene	Functional aberration of vital systems in the body like the reproductive, immune, nervous, endocrine, cardiovascular, and respiratory systems. Decrease in HB, platelet count, and WBC count	Haji Bahadar, Sara Mostafalou, Mohammad Abdollahi. Current understandings and perspectives on non-cancer health effects of benzene: a global concern, Toxicology and Applied Pharmacology, Volume 276, Issue 2, 2014, Pages 83–94, https://doi.org/10.1016/j.taap.2014.02.012.
	Neurological abnormalities (atrophy of lower extremities and neuropathy of upper extremities)	Aynur Baslo, Muzaffer Aksoy. Neurological abnormalities in chronic benzene poisoning. A study of six patients with aplastic anemia and two with preleukemia. Environmental Research, Volume 27, Issue 2, 1982, 457–465. https://doi.org/10.1016/0013-9351(82)90100-1.
	Increased CVD risk and deficits in circulating angiogenic cells in both smokers and nonsmokers	Abplanalp W, DeJarnett N, Riggs DW, Conklin DJ, McCracken JP, et al. (2017) Benzene exposure is associated with cardiovascular disease risk. PLOS ONE 12(9): e0183602. https://doi.org/10.1371/journal.pone.0183602
	Pancytopenia. Continued exposure to benzene can also result in aplastic anemia or leukemia. Myalgia, produces changes in the levels of antibodies in the blood, and decreases the numbers of mature B- and T-lymphocytes produced in the bone marrow, spleen, and thymus. Drowsiness, dizziness, headache, vertigo, tremor, delirium, and loss of consciousness. Global atrophy of lower extremities and distal neuropathy of upper extremities. Difficulty sleeping and complaints of memory loss	Toxicological profile for benzene. Atlanta (GA): Agency for Toxic Substances and Disease Registry (US); 2007 Aug. https://www.ncbi.nlm.nih.gov/books/NBK591293/

(continued)

Table 1 (continued)

Chemical carcinogens	Nonmalignant disorders/diseases	Sources
Benzidine	Immunologic, neurologic, reproductive, developmental, genotoxic, dermal sensitization, allergic contact dermatitis, decrease in liver and kidney body weight, an increase in spleen weight, swelling of the liver, and blood in the urine	CHOUDHARY, G. Human health perspectives on environmental exposure to benzidine: a review. **Chemosphere**, *[s. l.]*, v. 32, n. 2, p. 267–291, 1996. https://doi.org/10.1016/0045-6535(95)00338-X. Disponível em: https://ezproxy.nb.rs:4528/linkprocessor/plink?id=09386ed3-4668-3ea0-b797-2b78d8229770. Acesso em: 10 out. 2024.
Benzo(a)pyrene	Toxicological effects in the vessel wall cells, atherogenic effect, abdominal aortic aneurysm, myocardial injury, hypertension	Fu C, Li Y, Xi H, Niu Z, Chen N, Wang R, Yan Y, Gan X, Wang M, Zhang W, Zhang Y and Lv P (2022) Benzo(a)pyrene and cardiovascular diseases: an overview of pre-clinical studies focused on the underlying molecular mechanism. *Front. Nutr.* 9:978475. https://doi.org/10.3389/fnut.2022.978475
	Leads to a prolonged gestation period, earlier mean menopausal age, altered ovarian steroidogenesis, and ovarian reserve depletion, neurotoxic disorders	Bukowska, B.; Mokra, K.; Michałowicz, J. Benzo[a]pyrene—environmental occurrence, human exposure, and mechanisms of toxicity. *Int. J. Mol. Sci.* **2022**, *23*, 6348. https://doi.org/10.3390/ijms23116348
1,3-Butadiene	Exposure to BD has been associated with leukemia, cardiovascular disease, and possibly reproductive effects, autism, and asthma in children	Chen WQ, Zhang XY. 1,3-Butadiene: a ubiquitous environmental mutagen and its associations with diseases. Genes Environ. 2022 Jan 10;44(1):3. https://doi.org/10.1186/s41021-021-00233-y. PMID: 35012685; PMCID: PMC8744311.
	Emphysema and cardiovascular diseases (chronic rheumatic and atherosclerotic heart disease)	Huy, L. N., Lee, S. C. & Zhang, Z. Human cancer risk estimation for 1, 3-butadiene: an assessment of personal exposure and different microenvironments. *Sci. Total Environ.* **616**, 1599–1611 (2018).
Vinyl chloride	Induces chromosomal damage	Wei Wang, Yu-Lan Qiu, Jie Jiao, Jing Liu, Fang Ji , Wen-Bin Miao, Yiliang Zhu, Zhao-Lin Xia. Genotoxicity in vinyl chloride-exposed workers and its implication for occupational exposure limit. Am. J. Ind. Med. 54:800–810, 2011. © 2011 Wiley-Liss, Inc.
	Fibrosis, cirrhosis, and steatohepatitis in vinyl chloride workers following chronic-duration inhalation exposure. Immunological effects are increase in circulating immune complexes, immunoglobulins, complement factors, and levels of inflammatory cytokines	Toxicological profile for vinyl chloride. Atlanta (GA): Agency for Toxic Substances and Disease Registry (US); 2024 Jan. CHAPTER 2, HEALTH EFFECTS. Available from: https://www.ncbi.nlm.nih.gov/books/NBK601943/
	"Vinyl chloride disease," which is characterized by Raynaud's phenomenon (blanched fingers and numbness and discomfort are experienced upon exposure to the cold), changes in the bones at the end of the fingers, joint and muscle pain, and scleroderma-like skin changes (thickening of the skin, decreased elasticity, and slight edema) CNS effects (including dizziness, drowsiness, fatigue, headache, visual and/or hearing disturbances, memory loss, and sleep disturbances) as well as peripheral nervous system symptoms (peripheral neuropathy, tingling, numbness, weakness, and pain in fingers) have also been reported in workers exposed to vinyl chloride	U.S. Department of Health and Human Services. ATSDR. Toxicological profile for vinyl chloride. January 2024.

1,2-Dichloropropane Protecting against noncancer lesions expected to protect against cancer	Impaired kidney function, tubular necrosis, and acute kidney failure. Allergic contact dermatitis, severe CNS depression, and coma have been reported in cases of accidental or intentional ingestion or intentional inhalation abuse, altered serum liver enzymes, impaired liver function, toxic hepatitis, hepatic necrosis, and liver failure. Hemolytic anemia as well as incidences of disseminated intravascular coagulation	U.S. Department of Health and Human Services. ATSDR. Toxicological profile for 1,2-dichloropropane. November 2021.
	Hemolytic anemia	Health Based Guidance for Water Health Risk Assessment Unit, Environmental Health Division 651-201-4899. Adopted as Rule: November 2023, Toxicological summary for: 1,2-dichloropropane
Ethylene oxide	Neuropathy, weakness in extremities, impaired hand-eye coordination, cognitive dysfunction, memory loss, headache, and lethargy were reported among workers exposed to ethylene oxide for various durations. Sural nerve biopsies revealed axonal degeneration and regeneration in two studies. Cataracts and corneal burns.	Toxicological profile for ethylene oxide. Atlanta (GA): Agency for Toxic Substances and Disease Registry (US); 2022 Aug. Available from: https://www.ncbi.nlm.nih.gov/books/NBK589517/
	Irritation of the eyes, skin, and respiratory passages and effects to the nervous system (e.g., headache, nausea, memory loss)	*Lake County, Illinois sent this bulletin at 06/26/2024.* Ethylene oxide health risks information for clinicians. https://content.govdelivery.com/bulletins/gd/ILLAKE-3a50f36?wgt_ref=ILLAKE_WIDGET_752
Hexachlorocyclohexane (HCH)	Type 2 diabetes, endometriosis	Rincón-Rubio, A., Mérida-Ortega, Á., Ugalde-Resano, R. *et al.* Carcinogenic, non-carcinogenic risk, and attributable cases to organochlorine pesticide exposure in women from Northern Mexico. *Environ Monit Assess* 196, 421 (2024). https://doi.org/10.1007/s10661-024-12584-4
	Dermatologic, neurologic, reproductive disorders	Non-cancer health effects of pesticides. M. Sanborn, K.J. Kerr, L.H. Sanin, D.C. Cole, K.L. Bassil, C. Vakil. Canadian Family Physician Oct 2007, 53 (10) 1712–1720
4,4′-Methylenebis(2-chloroaniline)	Methemoglobinemia; high or repeated exposure may affect the kidneys	IARC Monographs on the Identification of Carcinogenic Hazards to Humans, No. 127. IARC Working Group on the Identification of Carcinogenic Hazards to Humans. Lyon (FR): International Agency for Research on Cancer; 2021.
2-Naphthylamine	Ischemic heart diseases and cerebrovascular disease and nonmalignant respiratory diseases (bronchitis)	Broekhuizen, Pieter. Airborne release of tyre wear particles—update 2024. February 2024. https://doi.org/10.13140/RG.2.2.19335.57760

(continued)

Table 1 (continued)

Chemical carcinogens	Nonmalignant disorders/diseases	Sources
Ortho-toluidine	Methemoglobinemia, damage to the nervous system, damage to the kidneys	New Jersey Department of Health. o-toluidine—hazardous substance fact sheet. https://nj.gov/health/eoh/rtkweb/documents/fs/1442.pdf
	Anemia, anorexia, weight loss, skin lesions, central nervous system depression, cyanosis, and methemoglobinemia	U.S. Environmental Protection Agency. 2-Methylaniline (o-Toluidine). https://www.epa.gov/sites/default/files/2016-09/documents/o-toluidine.pdf
Pentachlorophenol	Chronic health effects from long-term exposure to penta include impairment of the immune system, interference with reproduction, birth defects, and hormonal problems	Beyond Pesticides/National Coalition Against the Misuse of Pesticides (NCAMP). "Just how hazardous is pentachlorophenol?" https://www.beyondpesticides.org/assets/media/documents/wood/pubs/pole_pollution/Pole_report_no_app.pdf
	Body weight reduction, respiratory challenges, cardiovascular diseases, gastrointestinal problems, hematological, musculoskeletal, hepatic, renal, endocrine, immunological, neurological, and other noncancer diseases	Emenike C.U., He Q., Koushika K. Pentachlorophenol and its effect on different environmental matrices: the need for an alternative wood preservative. *Sustain Earth Reviews* **7**, 22 (2024). https://doi.org/10.1186/s42055-024-00090-x
	Chronic high-dose occupational exposure to pentachlorophenol causes inflammation of the upper respiratory tract and bronchitis. Increased risk of death from chronic obstructive pulmonary disease. Hyperthermia and tachycardia. Aplastic anemia, pure red blood cell aplasia, or severe pancytopenia with abnormal marrow. Increases in liver weight, hepatocellular hypertrophy, hepatocellular degeneration and necrosis, and chronic inflammation. Metabolic acidosis, proteinuria, and increased blood urea nitrogen; mild renal tubular degeneration; impaired glomerular filtration; chloracne, characterized by extensive cysts and pus-forming abscesses on the face, chest, abdomen, and proximal part of the extremities; neurotoxicity: an increase in subjective symptoms (increased fatigue, distractibility, attenuated motivation, and depressed mood) and impaired performance on several objective tests of neurobehavioral performance (paired-associated learning with a distracting condition, verbal memory test with distraction, visual short-term memory, and incidental learning of visual objects). Intermittent delirium and convulsions. Habitual abortion, unexplained infertility, menstrual disorders, or the onset of menopause	Atlanta (GA): Agency for Toxic Substances and Disease Registry (US); 2022 Apr. Toxicological Profile for Pentachlorophenol.

Polychlorinated biphenyls (PHBs) The different health effects of PCBs may be interrelated, as alterations in one system may have significant implications for the other systems of the body.	Suppress the immune system, learning deficits and changes in activity, neurobehavioral effects, decreased thyroid hormone levels, dermal and ocular effects, elevations in blood pressure, serum triglyceride, and serum cholesterol	US EPA. Health Effects| Polychlorinated Biphenyls (PCBs)| Wastes | http://www.epa.gov/epawaste/hazard/tsd/pcbs/pubs/effects.htm Last updated on Tuesday, April 03, 2012
	Diabetes mellitus and heart disease	Kashima, S., Yorifuji, T., Tsuda, T. *et al.* Cancer and non-cancer excess mortality resulting from mixed exposure to polychlorinated biphenyls and polychlorinated dibenzofurans from contaminated rice oil: "*Yusho*". *Int Arch Occup Environ Health* **88**, 419–430 (2015). https://doi.org/10.1007/s00420-014-0966-1
	Hypertension Ischemic heart disease (including myocardial infarction) Cerebrovascular disease (including stroke), chloracne Abnormal pigmentation, eczema, hyperkeratosis Nail deformities, developmental weight and size (early life), thyroid function, cirrhosis and steatosis Serum biomarkers of liver function disorders Cholesterol/triglyceride levels, immune suppression (including susceptibility to infection, antigen-specific antibody responses, WBC function) Atopy (including allergies/asthma), glucose homeostasis (including IR, IGT/prediabetes, type 2 diabetes mellitus, gestational diabetes), bone density/strength Dental abnormalities (including enamel defects and dental caries), cognitive function Attention, impulse control, externalizing and internalizing behaviors Executive function Motor function/development *Following developmental exposures:* Social cognition and behavior Auditory function, ocular swelling and irritation (including periorbital edema, ocular discharge, meibomian gland enlargement, conjunctivitis), sex hormone levels Fertility Sperm/semen parameters Gestation length (including preterm birth) Endometriosis Pubertal development Endpoints associated with testicular dysgenesis syndrome (including anogenital distance, hypospadias, cryptorchidism, sex ratio), pulmonary health and function (including chest radiography, spirometry, respiratory sounds, sputum analysis)	Laura M. Carlson, Krista Christensen, Sharon K. Sagiv, Pradeep Rajan, Carolyn R. Klocke, Pamela J. Lein, Evan Coffman, Rachel M. Shaffer, Erin E. Yost, Xabier Arzuaga, Pam Factor-Litvak, Alexander Sergeev, Michal Toborek, Michael S. Bloom, Joanne Trgovcich, Todd A. Jusko, Larry Robertson, John D. Meeker, Aileen F. Keating, Robyn Blain, Raquel A. Silva, Samantha Snow, Cynthia Lin, Kelly Shipkowski, Brandall Ingle, Geniece M. Lehmann, A systematic evidence map for the evaluation of noncancer health effects and exposures to polychlorinated biphenyl mixtures, Environmental Research, Volume 220, 2023, 115148, https://doi.org/10.1016/j.envres.2022.115148.

(continued)

Table 1 (continued)

Chemical carcinogens	Nonmalignant disorders/diseases	Sources
PAHs	Reduced lung function, exacerbation of asthma, and increased rates of obstructive lung diseases and ischemia, myocardial infarction, stroke, elevated blood pressure, peripheral arterial disease, heart rate variability, atherosclerosis and thrombosis.	Human health effects of polycyclic aromatic hydrocarbons as ambient air pollutants: report of the Working Group on Polycyclic Aromatic Hydrocarbons of the Joint Task Force on the Health Aspects of Air Pollution. Copenhagen: WHO Regional Office for Europe; 2021. Licence: CC BY-NC-SA 3.0 IGO.
	Cataracts, kidney and liver damage, and jaundice. Redness and inflammation of the skin. Breathing or swallowing large amounts of naphthalene can cause the breakdown of red blood cells and decreased immune function	Illinois Department of Public Health Division of Environmental Health 525 W. Jefferson St. Springfield, IL. POLYCYCLIC AROMATIC HYDROCARBONS (PAHs). http://www.idph.state.il.us/cancer/factsheets/polycyclicaromatichydrocarbons.htm
2,3,7,8-Tetrachlorodibenzo-para-dioxin	Chloracne, there are a variety of signs and symptoms (ranging from gastrointestinal disturbances to metabolic disorders) which accompany the appearance of the skin eruptions and persist for varying lengths of time	CDC. National Institute for Occupational Safety and Health. 2,3,7,8-Tetrachlorodibenzo-p-dioxin (TCDD, "dioxin"). **Current Intelligence Bulletin 40.** June 6, 2014.
	May damage the liver, can affect the nervous system with symptoms of weakness, personality and mood changes, pain in the legs and numbness; may decrease fertility in males and females	New Jersey Department of Health and Senior Services. 2,3,7,8-Tetrachlorodibenzo-para-dioxin. September 2002. https://nj.gov/health/eoh/rtkweb/documents/fs/1806.pdf
2,3,4,7,8-Pentachlorodibenzofuran	Anemia, more frequent lung infections, numbness, effects on the nervous system, mild changes in the liver defects in the progeny and injury to male or female reproductive function. Developmental effects. Chloracne; hyperpigmentation of the skin, nails, and gingivae; deformed nails; conjunctivitis; meibomian gland changes (enlargement, inflammation, hypersecretion of cheese-like material); and dark-colored pigmentation of the conjunctivae and eyelids	DHHS/ATSDR; Toxicological Profile for Chlorodibenzofurans p.43 (1994). Available from, as of September 19, 2003: https://www.atsdr.cdc.gov/toxprofiles/tp32.html DHHS/ATSDR; Toxicological Profile for Chlorodibenzofurans p. 36 (1994). Available from, as of September 17, 2003: https://www.atsdr.cdc.gov/toxprofiles/tp32.html

Trichlorethylene	Noncancer toxicity to the nervous system (dizziness, headaches, confusion, euphoria, facial numbness, and weakness), kidneys, liver, immune system, male reproductive system effects on the testes, epididymides, sperm, or hormone levels) and the developing embryo/fetus (fetal cardiac malformations), hepatotoxicity (jaundice; scleral icterus; elevated alanine transaminase [ALT], aspartate transaminase [AST], some bilirubin levels and hepatomegaly), nephrotoxicity(reduced glomerular filtration rate, elevated uric acid levels, and renal tubular injury), autoimmune disease, skin (exfoliative dermatitis, erythema multiforme, severe multiforme major, and bullosa epidermal necrolysis, including scleroderma and a specific type of generalized hypersensitivity disorder), cardiovascular (myocardial damage and congenital heart defects, as well as an increased risk of vascular embolism), gastrointestinal inflammation, ulcers, and damage	CDC. Agency for Toxic Substances and Disease Registry. September 9, 2022. https://www.atsdr.cdc.gov/csem/trichloroethylene/clinical_effects.html USA. EPA. Trichloroethylene. January 2000. https://www.epa.gov/sites/default/files/2016-09/documents/trichloroethylene.pdf Lifu Zhu, Xueqian Jia, Haibo Xie, Jiaxiang Zhang, Qixing Zhu, Trichloroethylene exposure, multi-organ injury, and potential mechanisms: A narrative review, Science of The Total Environment, Volume 946, 2024, 174029, https://doi.org/10.1016/j.scitotenv.2024.174029.

Appendix: General Questions to Ask the Patient

1. Do you take nutritional supplements (minerals, vitamins, elements)?   Yes   No

   How often do you take them:
   (a) Daily
   (b) Three times a week
   (c) Once a week or less often

   List what nutritional supplements you take: ……………………………………………… …………………………… …………………………………………………………………………………………………… ……………………………

2. How often do you stay in a smoking room for more than two hours?
   (a) Daily
   (b) Three times a week
   (c) Once a week or less often

3. Daily intake of tap water in liters: ……………………………………………………………… ……………………………

4. Daily intake of other liquids in liters (bottled water, juices, beer)…………………… …………………… …………………………………………………………………………………………………… …………………………… …………………………………………………………………………………………………… ……………………………

References

1. Radosavljevic V. Urinary markers/metabolites of exposure to chemical carcinogens—new possibilities in preventive oncology. Ecotoxicol Environ Saf. 2024; https://doi.org/10.1016/j.ecoenv.2023.115774.
2. WHO (IARC). Cancer today. 2024. https://gco.iarc.fr/today/en/dataviz/tables?mode=population. Accessed on 9 Aug 2024.
3. Siegel RL, Giaquinto AN, Jemal A. Cancer statistics, 2024. CA Cancer J Clin. 2024;4:12–49. https://doi.org/10.3322/caac.21820.
4. Zulpaite G, Zulpaite R, Vezelis A. Scrotal squamous cell carcinoma: a case report. J Surg Case Rep. 2023;3:1–3. https://doi.org/10.1093/jscr/rjad128.
5. American Cancer Society. Latest global cancer statistics. 2024. https://pressroom.cancer.org/GlobalCancerStatistics2024. Accessed 10 Aug 2024.
6. Radosavljević V. Urinarni markeri ekspozicije hemijskim kancerogenima—nove smernice u preventivnoj onkologiji (Urinary markers of exposure to chemical carcinogens—new guidelines in preventive oncology). Beograd: Medija centar „Odbrana"; 2024.

Human Exposure to Arsenic and Inorganic Arsenic Compounds

2.1 Overview

As in food products and ingredients is a concern because this metal is ubiquitous in the environment and, as such, can reach the food supply via accumulation in plants, animals, and water sources [1]. Many different varieties of *As* and *As* compounds exist naturally in the environment as metal ores in the Earth's crust and are also transported to different parts of the world by various natural cycles. For example, *As* in soil or in ores can be dissolved by rain such that the dissolved metals can enter river and groundwater systems and later the oceans and deposit as sediments. *As* may also be dispersed into the atmosphere along with water vapor and subsequently deposit elsewhere. *As* from the air and soil could be taken up by edible plants and taken up by fish in streams and oceans and come to the human diet [2]. Our task is to reduce or eliminate exposure of *As* in food, dietary supplements, and cosmetics [1]. Uses of arsenic today include pharmaceuticals, wood preservatives, agricultural chemicals, mining, metallurgical, glass, and semiconductor applications. Arsenic is the 20th most common element in the Earth's crust and is present in more than 200 mineral species. In the environment, it is mainly transmitted by water. The primary route of exposure of the general population to arsenic is through consumption of contaminated food or water [3, 4]. The highest concentrations of arsenic were found in seafood, meat, cereals, vegetables, fruit, and dairy products. Inorganic arsenic is the dominant form and is found in meat, poultry, dairy products, and grains, and organic arsenic (arsenobetaine) predominates in seafood, fruits, and vegetables [5–7]. In the US Total Diet Study, *As* was on the first place by representation among 11 prominent environmental contaminants, very dangerous to human health [8]. The major food group contributors to total arsenic exposure for the general US population were marine sources, which accounted for 69% of the total arsenic exposure, and grains, legumes, and seeds, which accounted for 20% [9–11]. Dietary exposure to arsenic may be an important source even when drinking water levels are low. In Korea, seaweed is consumed by itself as an ingredient of soup stock and processed foods. Thus, Korean dietary habits may be responsible for the increased urinary DMA levels and seaweed is also consumed in various other Asian countries such as Japan and China. Accordingly, urinary arsenic may be higher in East Asian countries than in Europe and the United States [12].

Inorganic arsenic was found at ng/g concentrations in most foods tested. In fruits and vegetables, inorganic arsenic accounted for approximately one-half of the total arsenic. In grains, sugars, and oil, inorganic arsenic accounted for approximately one-quarter of the total arsenic, while only a small fraction of the total was inorganic in meat, poultry, fish, and eggs [10]. The daily intake of total arsenic from food and drink is generally 20–300 µg. It is assumed that the daily inhalation intake can be about 20–200 ng in rural areas, 400–600 ng in cities without significant industrial arsenic emissions, about 1 µg/day in nonsmokers and in more polluted areas, and up to approximately 10 µg/day in smokers [6, 13]. In the Serbian market-basket study, *As* was detected in only four analyzed food items: canned fish (0.43 mg/kg), sausage (0.04 mg/kg), oil (0.03 mg/kg), and margarine (0.03 mg/kg). For adults the estimated intake of *As* through the studied foodstuffs was 21.89 µg/day [14].

Mechanism of inorganic As influence on blood pressure is still unclear [15]. Inorganic arsenic compounds cause lung, bladder, and skin cancer. Also, a positive association was observed between exposure to arsenic and inorganic arsenic compounds and cancer of the kidney, liver and prostate. Chronic exposure of humans to inorganic arsenic (InAs) has been associated with increased risk of cancer, disorders of the peripheral vasculature, diseases of the cardiovascular and cerebrovascular systems, hypertension, diabetes, and reproductive failure [3].

Urinary arsenic metabolites commonly used as indicators of recent exposure are total inorganic arsenic, arsenobetaine, methylarsonic acid (MAA), and dimethylarsinic acid (DMAA).

Appendix: Exposure Evaluation Questionnaire

1. Do you consume sweets additionally (in addition to regular meals) and how much in grams or teaspoons (coffee with sugar, added sugar to drinks—lemonade, diluted juices, cakes, cakes)? ....

....

....

....

2. Do you consume sweets with rice and how much—(a) several times a day, (b) once daily, (c) three times a week, and (d) once a week—and in what quantity in grams?..............................

3. Are the sweets you consume wrapped in foil? ....Yes   No.........

4. Do you consume extra (in addition to regular meals) and how much in pieces: carrots, cucumbers, onions (summer or winter salads)? ....
...........Yes...No

5. If the previous answer is Yes, how many times do you consume—(a) several times a day, (b) once a day, (c) three times a week, and (d) once a week—and in what quantity in pieces?................

6. Do you consume apple juice and how much—(a) several times a day, (b) once daily, (c) three times a week, and (d) once a week—and in what quantity in milliliters?...

7. Do you consume orange juice and how much—(a) several times a day, (b) once daily, (c) three times a week, and (d) once a week—and in what quantity in milliliters?............................

8. Do you consume peach juice and how much—(a) several times a day, (b) once daily, (c) three times a week, and (d) once a week—and in what quantity in milliliters?...

9. Are the juices you consume or any other type of food from Tetra Pak packaging?................

10. How often do you eat pastries—(a) several times a day, (b) once daily, (c) three times a week, and (d) once a week—and in what quantity in grams?................
....

11. How often do you eat bread and what kind—(a) several times a day and (b) once a day—and in what amount in grams?...
....

12. Do you consume seafood and/or fish?   Yes   No

13. If you consume seafood and/or fish, how often:
    (a) Daily
    (b) Three times a week
    (c) Once a week or less often

14. Do you consume sauces and which ones: Yes   No ....
....

15. If you consume sauces, how often:
    (a) Daily
    (b) Three times a week
    (c) Once a week or less often

References

1. Wong C, Roberts SM, Saab IN. Review of regulatory reference values and background levels for heavy metals in the human diet. Regul Toxicol Pharmacol. 2022; https://doi.org/10.1016/j.yrtph.2022.105122.

2. Tran NL, Barraj LM, Scrafford C, Bi X, Troxell T. Partitioning of dietary metal intake—a metal dietary exposure screening tool. Risk Anal. 2015;35:872–81.

3. Calderon RL, Hudgens E, Le XC, Schreinemachers D, Thomas DJ. Excretion of arsenic in urine as a function of exposure to arsenic in drinking water. Environ Health Perspect. 1999;107:663–7. http://ehpnetl.niehs.nib

4. Bae H-S, Ryu D-Y, Choi B-S, Park J-D. Urinary arsenic concentrations and their associated factors in Korean adults. Toxicol Res. 2013;29:137–42. https://doi.org/10.5487/TR.2013.29.2.137.

5. MacIntosh DL, Williams PL, Hunter DJ, Sampson LA, Morris SC, Willett WC, et al. Evaluation of a food frequency questionnaire-food composition approach for estimating dietary intake of inorganic arsenic and methylmercury. Cancer Epidemiol Biomarkers Prev. 1997;6:1043–50.

6. WHO. Air quality guidelines for Europe, European series, no. 91. 2nd ed. Copenhagen: WHO Regional Publications; 2000. https://iris.who.int/bitstream/handle/10665/107335/9789289013581-eng.pdf?sequence=1. Accessed 11 Aug 2024.

7. WHO. Arsenic and arsenic compounds, Environmental health criteria 224. 2nd ed. Geneva: World Health Organization, International Programme on Chemical Safety; 2001. https://iris.who.int/bitstream/10665/42366/1/WHO_EHC_224.pdf. Accessed 11 Aug 2024.

8. Macintosh DL, Spengler JD, Ozkaynak H, Tsai L-H, Ryan PB. Dietary exposures to selected metals and pesticides. Environ Health Perspect. 1996;104:202–9.

9. Jara EA, Winter CK. Dietary exposure to total and inorganic arsenic in the United States, 2006–2008. Food Contam. 2014; https://doi.org/10.1186/s40550-014-0003-x.

10. Schoof RA, Yost LJ, Eickhoff J, Crecelius EA, Cragin DW, Meacher DM, et al. A market basket survey of inorganic arsenic in food. Food Chem Toxicol. 1999;37:839–46.

11. Moschandreas DJ, Karuchit S, Berry MR, O'Rourke MK, Lo D, Lebowitz MD, Robertson G. Exposure apportionment: ranking food items by their contribution to dietary exposure. J Expo Sci Environ Epidemiol. 2002;12:233–43.

12. Lee JW, Lee CK, Moon CS, Choi IJ, Lee KJ, Yi S-M, et al. Korea National Survey for Environmental Pollutants in the Human Body 2008: heavy metals in the blood or urine of the Korean population. Int J Hyg Environ Health. 2012;215:449–57. https://doi.org/10.1016/j.ijheh.2012.01.002.

13. Radosavljević V. Urinarni markeri ekspozicije hemijskim kancerogenima—nove smernice u preventivnoj onkologiji (Urinary markers of exposure to chemical carcinogens—new guidelines in preventive oncology). Beograd: Medija centar „Odbrana"; 2024.

14. Škrbic B, Zivancev J, Mrmoš N. Concentrations of arsenic, cadmium and lead in selected foodstuffs from Serbian market basket: estimated intake by the population from the Serbia. Food Chem Toxicol. 2013;58:440–8. https://doi.org/10.1016/j.fct.2013.05.026.

15. Mizuno Y, Shimizu-Furusawa H, Konishi S, Inaoka T, Ahmad SA, Sekiyama M, et al. Associations between urinary heavy metal concentrations and blood pressure in residents of Asian countries. Environ Health Prev Med. 2021; https://doi.org/10.1186/s12199-021-01027-y.

3

3.1 Overview

The average amount of cadmium in the Earth's crust is 0.1–0.2 mg/kg. Natural levels of cadmium in ocean water are from <5 to 110 ng/l [1–3]. The main use of cadmium is for nickel-cadmium (Ni-Cd) batteries, pigments, glass, glazes, ceramics, rubber, enamels, paints for artists, pyrotechnics, coatings and plating (iron, steel, aluminum, and nonferrous metals), stabilizers for plastics, nonferrous metal alloys (copper, zinc, lead, tin, silver, and other precious metals), semiconductors and photovoltaic devices, automotive systems, military equipment, and marine/shore installations [4–6]. Ni-Cd batteries are widely used in the railway and aircraft industries, cordless power tools, mobile phones, portable computers, portable home appliances, and toys [2, 4]. Cadmium is also present as an impurity in fossil fuels (coal, oil, gas), cement, and phosphate fertilizers [7].

The average daily dietary intake of cadmium for the US population was estimated at 18.9 µg/day [6, 8]. The estimated average weekly dietary intake in the EU was 2.5 µg/kg body weight [9]. The food groups that contributed most to Cd intake were cereals and bread (34%), leafy vegetables (20%), potatoes (11%), legumes and nuts (7%), and stem/root vegetables (6%). The foods that contributed most to total Cd intake were lettuce (14%), spaghetti (8%), bread (7%), and potatoes (6%). Lettuce was the major Cd source for Caucasians and Blacks, whereas tortillas were the top source for Hispanics, and rice was the top contributor among other ethnic subgroups including Asians [10, 11]. The Cd content exceeded the maximum acceptable level among the fruit samples in frozen and frozen strawberries. In the case of vegetables, this result was observed in fresh beetroots, frozen carrot, fresh celery, and processed tomatoes [9, 12]. According Cd contents found in the Serbian market-basket study, the analyzed food items could be ordered as follows: paprika > chocolate > candy = canned fish > white bread > sugar > sausage > cookies > potatoes, followed by pasta, pate, other types of bread, mushrooms, onion, prunes, bacon, hot dog, and hake, whereas the lowest content was found in oil, milk,

V. Radosavljevic, *Assessing Human Exposure to Key Chemical Carcinogens*, https://doi.org/10.1007/978-3-031-84441-6_3

apple, wheat flour, and hard cheese samples [13]. In spite of some expectations urinary cadmium (Cd) levels did not show a strong association with residential district (rural/urban/coastal) or seafood consumption [14].

In Poland, cereals accounted for the largest share of the overall Cd intake, accounting for 30.2% and 39.6% of the total daily intake of Cd among women and men, respectively. Vegetables were the second major food group significantly contributing to Cd intake (17.4% and 21% among women and men, respectively), followed by sweets (11% and 9.25%), meat and meat products (10% and 9%), and potatoes (9.25% and 10.2%). The obtained results are fully in agreement with other data, pointing to cereals as the major contributors to the total dietary intake of Cd. According to the EFSA study, cereals were contributing to the total intake of Cd (26.9%), followed by vegetables (16%), starchy roots and tubers (13.2%), and potatoes (13.2%) [15]. Potato consumption contributed close to a third of exposure in Irish adults (30%) and remained fairly high in many surveys except in Italy, Spain, and France. The dietary intake of Cd with meat was especially high in Hungary (25%) and the Czech Republic (15%), while the contribution of fish was the highest among Spanish (31%) and Italian adults (23%). Cereals were found to be the major contributor to an overall Cd intake also in other European countries: Denmark (49%), France (35%), Spain (37.9%), and Serbia (53.8%). Outside Europe, cereals are also a dominant contributor to Cd intake in Chile (37.9%) or Asian countries, where Cd is mostly consumed with rice and vegetables, which is understandable if we consider the structure of food consumption in this region [16]. In the US Total Diet Study, Cd was on the second place by representation among 11 prominent environmental contaminants (after As), very dangerous to human health [17]. The mechanism of Cd influence on blood pressure is still unclear [18].

Cadmium and cadmium compounds cause lung cancer and positive associations with kidney, pancreatic, and prostate cancers have been observed [19]. Cadmium is not metabolized in the body and its urinary biomarker of exposure is also cadmium [20].

Appendix: Exposure Evaluation Questionnaire

1. Do you consume cereals (corn, wheat, oatmeal) and how often:
   (a) Several times every day
   (b) Once a day
   (c) Three times a week
   (d) Once a week and less often
   And in what quantity do you consume cereals?......................................
   ....

2. Do you consume paprika and how often:
   (a) Daily
   (b) Three times a week
   (c) Once a week or less often

3. Do you consume chocolate and how often:
   (a) Daily
   (b) Three times a week
   (c) Once a week or less often
4. Do you consume canned fish and how often:
   (a) Daily
   (b) Three times a week
   (c) Once a week or less often
5. Do you consume sugar and how often:
   (a) Several times every day
   (b) Once a day
   (c) Three times a week
   (d) Once a week or less often
   And how much sugar do you consume?...
   ....
6. Do you consume potatoes and how often:
   (a) Several times every day
   (b) Once a day
   (c) Three times a week
   (d) Once a week and less often
   And in what quantity do you consume potatoes?.................................
   ....
7. Do you consume raspberries and how often:
   (a) Several times every day
   (b) Once a day
   (c) Three times a week
   (d) Once a week and less often
   And in what quantity do you consume raspberries?.............................
   ....
8. Do you consume strawberries and how often:
   (a) Several times every day
   (b) Once a day
   (c) Three times a week
   (d) Once a week and less often
   And in what quantity do you consume strawberries?...........................
   ....
9. Do you consume beets and how often:
   (a) Several times every day
   (b) Once a day
   (c) Three times a week
   (d) Once a week and less often
   And in what quantity do you consume beets?......................................
   ....

10. Do you consume carrots and how often:
    (a) Several times every day
    (b) Once a day
    (c) Three times a week
    (d) Once a week and less often
        And in what quantity do you consume carrots?...........................
        ....

11. Do you consume tomatoes and how often:
    (a) Several times every day
    (b) Once a day
    (c) Three times a week
    (d) Once a week and less often
        And in what quantity do you consume tomatoes?....................
        ....

References

1. ATSDR. Draft toxicological profile for cadmium. Atlanta: US Department of Health and Human Services; 2008.
2. UNEP. Interim review of scientific information on cadmium. Geneva: United Nations Environment Program; 2008.
3. Wong C, Roberts SM, Saab IN. Review of regulatory reference values and background levels for heavy metals in the human diet. Regul Toxicol Pharmacol. 2022; https://doi.org/10.1016/j.yrtph.2022.105122.
4. USGS. Mineral commodity summaries, cadmium; 2008, p. 42–43.
5. International Cadmium Association. 2011. Available at http://www.cadmium.org
6. CDC. Third national report on human exposure to environmental chemicals. US Department of Health and Human Services, Public Health Services. Centers for Disease Control and Prevention (CDC); 2005. Available at http://www.cdc.gov/exposurereport/
7. Canada. Natural Resources Canada. Minerals and Metals Sector. Canadian minerals yearbook: 2007 review and outlook. Ottawa: Natural Resources Canada; 2009. p. c2009. https://publications.gc.ca/site/eng/347677/publication.html
8. Tran NL, Barraj LM, Scrafford C, Bi X, Troxell T. Partitioning of dietary metal intake—a metal dietary exposure screening tool. Risk Anal. 2015;35:872–81.
9. EFSA. Cadmium in food. Scientific opinion of the panel on contaminants in the food chain. EFSA J. 2009;980:1–139. https://efsa.onlinelibrary.wiley.com/doi/epdf/10.2903/j.efsa.2009.980
10. Kim K, Melough MM, Vance TM, Noh H, Koo SI, Chun OK. Dietary cadmium intake and sources in the US. Nutrients. 2019; https://doi.org/10.3390/nu11010002.
11. Moschandreas DJ, Karuchit S, Berry MR, O'Rourke MK, Lo D, Lebowitz MD, Robertson G. Exposure apportionment: ranking food items by their contribution to dietary exposure. J Expo Sci Environ Epidemiol. 2002;12:233–43.
12. Rusin M, Domagalska J, Rogala D, Razzaghi M, Szymala I. Concentration of cadmium and lead in vegetables and fruits. Sci Rep. 2021; https://doi.org/10.1038/s41598-021-91554-z.
13. Škrbic B, Zivancev J, Mrmoš N. Concentrations of arsenic, cadmium and lead in selected foodstuffs from Serbian market basket: estimated intake by the population from the Serbia. Food Chem Toxicol. 2013;58:440–8. https://doi.org/10.1016/j.fct.2013.05.026.

14. Lee JW, Lee CK, Moon CS, Choi IJ, Lee KJ, Yi S-M, et al. Korea National Survey for Environmental Pollutants in the Human Body 2008: heavy metals in the blood or urine of the Korean population. Int J Hyg Environ Health. 2012;215:449–57. https://doi.org/10.1016/j.ijheh.2012.01.002.
15. European Food Safety Authority. Cadmium dietary exposure in the European population. EFSA J. 2012; https://www.efsa.europa.eu/en/efsajournal/pub/2551
16. Koch W, Czop M, Iłowiecka K, Nawrocka A, Wiacek D. Dietary intake of toxic heavy metals with major groups of food products—results of analytical determinations. Nutrients. 2022; https://doi.org/10.3390/nu14081626.
17. Macintosh DL, Spengler JD, Ozkaynak H, Tsai L-H, Ryan PB. Dietary exposures to selected metals and pesticides. Environ Health Perspect. 1996;104:202–9.
18. Mizuno Y, Shimizu-Furusawa H, Konishi S, Inaoka T, Ahmad SA, Sekiyama M, et al. Associations between urinary heavy metal concentrations and blood pressure in residents of Asian countries. Environ Health Prev Med. 2021; https://doi.org/10.1186/s12199-021-01027-y.
19. Radosavljević V. Urinarni markeri ekspozicije hemijskim kancerogenima—nove smernice u preventivnoj onkologiji (Urinary markers of exposure to chemical carcinogens—new guidelines in preventive oncology). Beograd: Medija centar „Odbrana"; 2024.
20. Radosavljevic V. Urinary markers/metabolites of exposure to chemical carcinogens—new possibilities in preventive oncology. Ecotoxicol Environ Saf. 2024; https://doi.org/10.1016/j.ecoenv.2023.115774.

Human Exposure to Nickel

4

4.1 Overview

Because of its corrosion resistance, heat resistance, hardness, and strength, nickel is part of many alloys. It is used in electroplating, ceramics, and pigments and as an intermediate (catalyst, formation of other nickel compounds). Ferronickel is used to prepare steel. Stainless steels contain as much as 25–30% nickel. Nickel is widely distributed in nature and is found in animals, plants, and soil [1].

It is the 24th most abundant element and makes up about 0.008% of the Earth's crust. Fossil fuel combustion is the largest contributor to atmospheric nickel, accounting for 62% of global anthropogenic emissions in the 1980s [2, 3]. Intake of nickel through food and, to a lesser extent, drinking water is the primary route of exposure for the general nonsmoking population [4].

The highest mean concentrations of nickel were measured in beans, nuts, and cereals [5]. Although nickel concentrations vary depending on the type of food, average levels are generally in the range of 0.01–0.1 µg/g [6, 7]. The main foods contributing to the nickel daily intake of 130.92 µg/day (102.80–168–94 µg/day) are cereals, legumes, vegetables, fresh fruits, sweets, particularly leafy vegetables, tomatoes, citrus fruits, chocolate products, and coffee and tea [6].

Nickel and nickel metal compounds cause lung, nasal cavity, and paranasal sinus cancer [8]. Soluble nickel compounds are rapidly absorbed through the lungs and excreted in the urine. In analytical papers, no one mentions metabolites, but they are determined as elements after destroying samples and releasing them from complexes with proteins where they are bound.

© The Author(s), under exclusive license to Springer Nature
Switzerland AG 2025
V. Radosavljevic, *Assessing Human Exposure to Key Chemical Carcinogens*,
https://doi.org/10.1007/978-3-031-84441-6_4

Appendix: Exposure Evaluation Questionnaire

1. Do you consume milk and dairy products (yogurt, sour milk, cheeses) and how often:
   (a) Several times every day
   (b) Once a day
   (c) Three times a week
   (d) Once a week and less often
   And in what quantity do you consume milk and milk products (specify which ones)?......................................
   ....
   ....

2. Do you consume meat and meat products (cured meat products) and how often:
   (a) Several times every day
   (b) Once a day
   (c) Three times a week
   (d) Once a week and less often
   And in what quantity do you consume meat and meat products (specify which ones)?......................................
   ....
   ....

3. Do you consume leafy vegetables and their products (lettuce, cabbage, kale, Swiss chard) and how often:
   (a) Several times every day
   (b) Once a day
   (c) Three times a week
   (d) Once a week and less often
   And in what quantity do you consume them (specify which leafy vegetables)?......................................
   ....
   ....

4. Do you consume legumes and their products (peas, green beans, beans) and how often:
   (a) Several times every day
   (b) Once a day
   (c) Three times a week
   (d) Once a week and less often
   And in what quantity do you consume them (specify which leguminous vegetables)?......................................
   ....
   ....

5. Do you consume other vegetables and products from other types of vegetables (fresh, canned, frozen, pasteurized) and how often:
   (a) Several times every day
   (b) Once a day
   (c) Three times a week
   (d) Once a week and less often
   And in what quantity do you consume vegetables and vegetable products (specify which ones)?....................................
   ....
   ....

6. Do you consume nuts and their products (walnuts, hazelnuts, almonds, peanuts, etc.) and how often:
   (a) Several times every day
   (b) Once a day
   (c) Three times a week
   (d) Once a week and less often
   And in what quantity do you consume nuts and products thereof (specify which ones)?.........................
   ....
   ....

7. Do you consume other fruits and other fruit products (fresh, canned, frozen, pasteurized) and how often:
   (a) Several times every day
   (b) Once a day
   (c) Three times a week
   (d) Once a week and less often
   And in what quantity do you consume fruit and fruit products (specify which ones)?...
   ....
   ....

8. Do you use oral contraceptives: Yes   No
9. If the previous answer is Yes, state which contraceptives you use and how often?
   ....
   ....

References

1. Barbante C, Boutron C, Moreau A-L, et al. Seasonal variations in nickel and vanadium in Mont Blanc snow and ice dated from the 1960s and 1990s. J Environ Monit. 2002;4:960–6.
2. ATSDR. Toxicological profile for nickel. Atlanta: US Public Health Service, Agency for Toxic Substances and Disease Registry; 2005.
3. OSHA; Occupational Safety and Health Administration. Department of Labor. Occupational exposure to hexavalent chromium. Final rule. Fed Regist. 2006;71:10099–385.

4. Moschandreas DJ, Karuchit S, Berry MR, O'Rourke MK, Lo D, Lebowitz MD, Robertson G. Exposure apportionment: ranking food items by their contribution to dietary exposure. J Expo Sci Environ Epidemiol. 2002;12:233–43.
5. Koch W, Czop M, Iłowiecka K, Nawrocka A, Wiacek D. Dietary intake of toxic heavy metals with major groups of food products—results of analytical determinations. Nutrients. 2022; https://doi.org/10.3390/nu14081626.
6. Filippini T, Tancredi S, Malagoli C, Malavolti M, Bargellini A, Vescovi L, et al. Dietary estimated intake of trace elements: risk assessment in an Italian population. Expo Health. 2020;12:641–55. https://doi.org/10.1007/s12403-019-00324-w.
7. Pearson AJ, Ashmore E. Risk assessment of antimony, barium, beryllium, boron, bromine, lithium, nickel, strontium, thallium and uranium concentrations in the New Zealand diet. Food Addit Contam Part A. 2020;37:451–64. https://doi.org/10.1080/19440049.2019.1704445.
8. Radosavljević V. Urinarni markeri ekspozicije hemijskim kancerogenima—nove smernice u preventivnoj onkologiji (Urinary markers of exposure to chemical carcinogens—new guidelines in preventive oncology). Beograd: Medija centar „Odbrana"; 2024.

Human Exposure to Beryllium

5

5.1   Overview

Beryllium is the 44th most abundant element in the Earth's crust and is released into the environment as a result of natural and anthropogenic activities [1–3]. About 50 minerals containing beryllium have been identified. The average amount of beryllium on Earth is 2–5.0 µg/kg [4, 5]. Bauxite, from which aluminum is obtained, can contain varying degrees of beryllium [6].

The main anthropogenic source of atmospheric beryllium is the burning of coal and fuel oil, and smaller sources are burning of waste, beryllium alloys, use of chemicals, and burning of solid rocket fuel [2, 7, 8]. Beryllium is ubiquitous and is used in metallic [1, 9] form, beryllium oxide alloys, and ceramics. Looking at its use, one should consider reducing exposure or finding a replacement. It is used in aerospace (altimeters, braking systems, engines, precision tools, solid propellant additives, satellite optical system mirror components, gyroscopes), automotive (air bag sensors, antilock systems, steering linkage springs), biomedicine (dental crowns, medical laser components, X-ray tube windows), defense (heat shields, missile guidance systems, nuclear reactor components, advanced surveillance satellites, and radar systems), energy and electronics (heat exchanger tubes, microwave devices, relays and switches), fire prevention (non-sparking tools in oil exploration equipment, sprinkler system springs), consumer products (camera shutters, computer disks, pencil clips), production of plastics (plastic injection molds), sporting goods (golf clubs, fishing rods, natural and artificial precious stones), and telecommunications (components for mobile phones, electronic and electrical connectors, housings for underwater repeaters) [1, 10–12]. Beryllium oxide is suitable for the production or protection of materials used at high temperatures in corrosive environments (it has ceramic properties).

In nonoccupationally exposed population, ingestion through foods and beverages is the main route of exposure. We found higher beryllium concentration in legumes, dry fruits, and sweet products, with also substantial content in all cereal

© The Author(s), under exclusive license to Springer Nature
Switzerland AG 2025
V. Radosavljevic, *Assessing Human Exposure to Key Chemical Carcinogens*,
https://doi.org/10.1007/978-3-031-84441-6_5

products but rice, leafy vegetables, red wine, and chocolate and biscuits/dry cakes. Beryllium daily intake is of 0.24 µg/day (IQR 0.18–0.32 µg/day) with main contribution from leafy vegetables, cereals (pasta and bread), beverages (particularly wine), and citrus fruits [13, 14], as well as in (below 100 µg/kg of dry weight) bananas, beans, cane sugar, coriander, dill, peas, green pepper, lettuce, mushrooms, parsley, pears, potatoes, rice, and pumpkins [15].

Beryllium and beryllium compounds cause cancerous diseases. Beryllium was detected in granulomas associated with chronic beryllium disease (CBD) in exposed workers for an average of several years. This indicates that beryllium is retained in granulomatous lesions for a long period of time in exposed humans. Inflammatory processes associated with the development of acute or chronic beryllium disease contribute to the development of lung cancer [16]. In analytical papers, no one mentions metabolites, but they are determined as elements after destroying samples and releasing them from complexes with proteins where they are bound.

Appendix: Exposure Evaluation Questionnaire

1. Do you consume bananas and how often:
   (a) Several times every day
   (b) Once a day
   (c) Three times a week
   (d) Once a week or less often
       And in what quantity do you consume bananas?......................................
   ....
2. Do you consume mushrooms and how often:
   (a) Several times every day
   (b) Once a day
   (c) Three times a week
   (d) Once a week or less often
       And in what quantity do you consume mushrooms?........................
   ....
3. Do you consume pears and how often:
   (a) Several times every day
   (b) Once a day
   (c) Three times a week
   (d) Once a week or less often
       And in what quantity do you consume pears?..
   ....

4. Do you consume pumpkins and how often:
   (a) Several times every day
   (b) Once a day
   (c) Three times a week
   (d) Once a week and less often
       And in what quantity do you consume pumpkins?..................................
   ....
5. Do you consume tomato juice and how often:
   (a) Several times every day
   (b) Once a day
   (c) Three times a week
   (d) Once a week and less often
       And how much tomato juice do you consume? ....
       .
6. Do you consume lemon or lemon juice (lemonade) and how often:
   (a) Several times every day
   (b) Once a day
   (c) Three times a week
   (d) Once a week or less often
       And in what quantity do you consume lemon or lemon juice
   (lemonade)?....................................

References

1. WHO. Beryllium. Environ Health Criteria; 1990. p. 106.
2. ATSDR. Toxicological profile for beryllium (US NTIS PB2003–100135). Atlanta: US Public Health Service, Agency for Toxic Substances and Disease Registry; 2002. Available at http://www.atsdr.cdc.gov/toxprofiles/tp4.pdf
3. Taylor TP, Ding M, Ehler DS, et al. Beryllium in the environment: a review. J Environ Sci Health A Tox Hazard Subst Environ Eng. 2003;38:439–69.
4. IARC. Beryllium, cadmium, mercury, and exposures in the glass manufacturing industry. IARC Monogr Eval Carcinog Risks Hum. 1993;58:1–415.
5. Jakubowski M, Palczynski C. Beryllium. In: Handbook on the toxicology of metals. 3rd ed. Academic; 2007. p. 415–31.
6. Taiwo OA, Slade MD, Cantley LF, et al. Beryllium sensitization in aluminum smelter workers. J Occup Environ Med. 2008;50:157–62.
7. WHO. Beryllium and beryllium compounds. Concise international chemical assessment, 32. Geneva: International Programme on Chemical Safety; 2001.
8. Kolanz ME. Introduction to beryllium: uses, regulatory history, and disease. Appl Occup Environ Hyg. 2001;16:559–67.
9. Petzow G, Fritz Aldinger WC, Jönsson S, Preuss OP. Beryllium and beryllium compounds. In: Gerhartz W, Yamamoto YS, Campbell FT, et al., editors. Ullmann's encyclopedia of industrial chemistry, vol. A4. 5th ed. Weinheim: VCH Verlagsgesellschaft; 1985. p. 11–33.
10. Petzow G, Fritz Aldinger WC, Jönsson S, et al. Beryllium and beryllium compounds. In: Ullmann's encyclopedia of industrial chemistry. 7th ed. Weinheim: VCH Verlagsgesellschaft; 2007. p. 1–28. [Online edition].
11. Kreiss K, Day GA, Schuler CR. Beryllium: a modern industrial hazard. Annu Rev Public Health. 2007;28:259–77.

12. Kaczynski DJ. Beryllium compounds. In: Kirk Othmer encyclopedia of chemical technology, vol. 3. 5th ed. New York: Wiley; 2004. p. 661–8. [Online version].
13. Filippini T, Tancredi S, Malagoli C, Malavolti M, Bargellini A, Vescovi L, et al. Dietary estimated intake of trace elements: risk assessment in an Italian population. Expo Health. 2020;12:641–55. https://doi.org/10.1007/s12403-019-00324-w.
14. Pearson AJ, Ashmore E. Risk assessment of antimony, barium, beryllium, boron, bromine, lithium, nickel, strontium, thallium and uranium concentrations in the New Zealand diet. Food Addit Contam Part A. 2020;37:451–64. https://doi.org/10.1080/19440049.2019.1704445.
15. Vaessen HAMG, Szteke B. Beryllium in food and drinking water: a summary of available knowledge. Food Addit Contam. 2000;17:149–59. https://doi.org/10.1080/026520300283504.
16. Radosavljević V. Urinarni markeri ekspozicije hemijskim kancerogenima—nove smernice u preventivnoj onkologiji (Urinary markers of exposure to chemical carcinogens—new guidelines in preventive oncology). Beograd: Medija centar „Odbrana“; 2024.

Human Exposure to Hexavalent Chromium

6.1 Overview

Chromium (VI) is found naturally in the Earth's crust, although it is mainly emitted into the environment as a result of anthropogenic activities [1]. There are two naturally occurring chromium (VI) compounds—lead chromate (crocoite) and potassium dichromate (lopesite) [2].

The arithmetic mean concentration of total chromium in the air (urban, suburban, and rural) was within ng/m^3 [3]. It was surprising that nearly 40% of municipal drinking water sources in California, USA, had chromium (VI) levels greater than 1 µg/l and average concentrations in the Canadian and US drinking water supplies ranging from 0.2 to 2 µg Cr(VI)/L [3]. The concentration of total chromium (geometric mean) was 37.0 mg/kg (range, 1.0–2000 mg/kg) based on 1319 samples collected in US soil [3].

Most of the chromium that is ingested through food is chromium (III) [6, 7]. Tobacco smoke contains chromium (VI). Indoor air polluted by cigarette smoke contains tens or even hundreds of times higher concentrations of chromium (VI) than outdoor air.

Chromium (VI) compounds are widely used in pigments for textile dyes (ammonium dichromate, potassium chromate, sodium chromate), inks and plastics (potassium dichromate, sodium chromate, lead chromate, zinc chromate, barium chromate, calcium chromate), corrosion inhibitors (barium chromate, calcium chromate, sodium chromate), wood preservatives (chromium trioxide), metal finishing, chrome plating (chromium trioxide), and leather tanning (ammonium dichromate) [2, 8].

Chromium (VI) can be present as an impurity in cement, so it is a ubiquitous carcinogen. Living or working near anthropogenic sources of chromium (VI) exposes people to breathing contaminated air or drinking contaminated water [4].

The main routes of occupational exposure are inhalation of dust, mist, or smoke and dermal contact with products containing chromium. Industries and occupations

V. Radosavljevic, *Assessing Human Exposure to Key Chemical Carcinogens*, https://doi.org/10.1007/978-3-031-84441-6_6

in which exposure to chromium (VI) is high are welding, production and use of metals and alloys containing chromium (stainless steels, steels with a high chromium content), galvanization, and production and use of pigments, dyes (application in the aviation industry), catalysts, chromic acid, tanning agents, and pesticides [1, 2]. CAREX (CARcinogen EXPosure) Canada (2011) estimated that 83,000 Canadians were occupationally exposed to chromium (VI) compounds [9].

Chromium (VI) compounds cause lung cancer, and very weak positive associations have been documented between exposure to chromium (VI) compounds and cancers of the stomach, nose, and nasal sinuses [2]. In analytical papers, no one mentions metabolites, but they are determined as elements after destroying samples and releasing them from complexes with proteins where they are bound.

Appendix: Exposure Evaluation Questionnaire

1. Have you worked in the wood protection industry or in the wood industry in general, the paint and pigment industry, metal chroming industry, leather industry, alloy industry, or paper and pulp industry?
2. If you have worked in any of the abovementioned industries, please indicate how long you have worked there and in which jobs exactly..
....
....
....
....
....
3. If you lived near any of the abovementioned industries, state how long you lived there and whether you visited the mentioned industries ....
....
....
....
4. Did you consume vegetables, beans, and cereals in larger quantities than usual (when and how much)?..
....
....
5. Do you suffer from asthma or anemia (when did your illness start)?...................
....
....
....
6. In the last week, have you noticed irritation of the nose, eyes, or skin?...............
....

Further Readings

1. Mohanty S, Benya A, Hota S, Kumar MS, Singh S. Ecotoxicity of hexavalent chromium and its adverse impact on environment and human health in Sukinda Valley of India: a review on pollution and prevention strategies. J Environ Chem Ecotoxicol. 2023;5:46–54. https://doi.org/10.1016/j.enceco.2023.01.002.
2. IARC. Chromium, nickel and welding. IARC monographs on the evaluation of carcinogenic risks to humans; 1990. https://publications.iarc.fr/Book-And-Report-Series/Iarc-Monographs-On-The-Identification-Of-Carcinogenic-Hazards-To-Humans/Chromium-Nickel-And-Welding-1990
3. ATSDR. Chromium (TP-7). In: Toxicological profile. US Department of Health and Human Services, Agency for Toxic Substances and Disease Registry; 2000. p. 461.
4. Sedman RM, Beaumont J, McDonald TA, et al. Review of the evidence regarding the carcinogenicity of hexavalent chromium in drinking water. J Environ Sci Health C Environ Carcinog Ecotoxicol Rev. 2006;24:155–82.
5. Moffat I, Martinova N, Seidel C, Thompson CM. Hexavalent chromium in drinking water. J AWWA (Am Water Works Assoc). 2018;110:5.
6. EVM Expert Group on Vitamins and Minerals Secretariat. Review of chromium. UK: EVM/99/26. 2002. Revised Aug 2002. p. 25.
7. Moschandreas DJ, Karuchit S, Berry MR, O'Rourke MK, Lo D, Lebowitz MD, Robertson G. Exposure apportionment: ranking food items by their contribution to dietary exposure. J Expo Anal Environ Epidemiol. 2002;12:233–43.
8. Mondal MH, Begum W, Nasrollahzadeh M, Ghorbannezhad F, Antoniadi V, Levizou E, et al. A comprehensive review on chromium chemistry along with detection, speciation, extraction and remediation of hexavalent chromium in contemporary science and technology. Vietnam J Chem. 2021;59(6):711–32. https://doi.org/10.1002/vjch.202100048.
9. CAREX Canada. 2011. Available at http://www.carexcanada.ca/en/chromium_%28hexavalent%29/occupational_exposure_estimates/phase_2/

7.1 Overview

7.1.1 Exposure of the General Population

A. flavus is especially widespread in the tropics and its main hosts are corn, peanuts, and cotton seeds [1, 2]. Also, various spices sometimes contain aflatoxins, while nuts are less frequently contaminated. Almost all aflatoxins in staple foods such as corn are ubiquitous [3]. Due to the movement of agricultural products around the world, no region is free of aflatoxin [3–5]. Aflatoxins B1, B2, G1, and G2 can be collected in dust in food processing plants (cocoa, coffee, and spices) [6]. According to FAO data, aflatoxins contaminate a quarter of the world's crops annually. The temperature at which most aflatoxins are produced is 33 °C [7, 8].

The risk of hepatocellular carcinoma (HCC) is significantly increased for subjects with high urinary concentrations of aflatoxin metabolites [9–11]. Their urinary metabolites are aflatoxin-N7-guanine adducts in urine [12, 13].

Appendix: Exposure Evaluation Questionnaire

1. In the last few days, have you had nausea, unsteady gait, loss of appetite, lethargy, jaundice, stomach pain, swelling, or spontaneous bleeding? ....
....
....
....

© The Author(s), under exclusive license to Springer Nature
Switzerland AG 2025
V. Radosavljevic, *Assessing Human Exposure to Key Chemical Carcinogens*,
https://doi.org/10.1007/978-3-031-84441-6_7

2. Have you consumed nuts (Brazilian, Indian, European) in the last few days and how often:
   (a) Daily
   (b) Three times a week
   (c) Once a week or less often

3. Have you consumed seeds (rich in oil) in the last few days and how often:
   (a) Daily
   (b) Three times a week
   (c) Once a week or less often

4. If you consume corn and corn products, how often:
   (a) Daily
   (b) Three times a week
   (c) Once a week or less often

5. If you consume peanuts, pistachios, and/or hazelnuts, how often:
   (a) Daily
   (b) Three times a week
   (c) Once a week or less often

6. If you consume apricots, figs, mulberries, dates, and/or sugar from Chinese cane, how often:
   (a) Daily
   (b) Three times a week
   (c) Once a week or less often

7. If you consume rice and/or rice foods, how often:
   (a) Daily
   (b) Three times a week
   (c) Once a week or less often

8. If you consume pastries, how often:
   (a) Daily
   (b) Three times a week
   (c) Once a week or less often

9. If you consume soy and/or soy products, how often:
   (a) Daily
   (b) Three times a week
   (c) Once a week or less often

10. If you consume milk, yogurt, cheese, baby milk, powdered milk, flavored milk, and/or other dairy products, how often:
    (a) Daily
    (b) Three times a week
    (c) Once a week or less often

11. Do you consume any other cereals and how often:
    (a) Daily
    (b) Three times a week
    (c) Once a week or less often

References

1. Meneely JP, Kolawole O, Haughey SA, Miller SJ, Krska R, Elliott CT. The challenge of global aflatoxins legislation with a focus on peanuts and peanut products: a systematic review. Expo Health. 2023;15:467–87. https://doi.org/10.1007/s12403-022-00499-9.
2. Bhardwaj K, Meneely JP, Haughey SA, Dean M, Wall P, Zhang G, Baker B, Elliott CT. Risk assessments for the dietary intake aflatoxins in food: a systematic review (2016–2022). Food Control. 2023;149:109687.
3. Zahra N, Raza MH, Hafeez F, Saeed MK, Khan SA, Saeed A, Shahzad K. Impact of aflatoxins exposure on human health and its management strategies. LGU J Life Sci. 2023;7(2):156–72. https://doi.org/10.54692/lgujls.2023.0702258.
4. IARC. Some traditional herbal medicines, some mycotoxins, naphthalene and styrene. IARC Monogr Eval Carcinog Risks Hum. 2002;82:1–556.
5. Qin M, Cheng L, Li Y, Tang X, Gan Y, Zhao J, Luo S, Zhang H, Zhang L, Chen J, Huo J. Disease burden contributed by dietary exposure to aflatoxins in a mountainous city in Southwest China. Front Microbiol. 2023;14:1215428. https://doi.org/10.3389/fmicb.2023.1215428.
6. Brera C, Caputi R, Miraglia M, et al. Exposure assessment to mycotoxins in workplaces: aflatoxins and ochratoxin A occurrence in airborne dusts and human sera. Microchem J. 2002;73:167–73.
7. Ismail AM, Raza MH, Zahra N, Ahmad R, Sajjad Y, Khan SA. Aflatoxins in wheat grains: detection and detoxification through chemical, physical, and biological means. Life. 2024;14:535. https://doi.org/10.3390/life14040535.
8. Alameri MM, Kong AS, Aljaafari MN, Ali HA, Eid K, Sallagi MA, Cheng WH, Abushelaibi A, Lim SE, Loh JY, Lai KS. Aflatoxin contamination: an overview on health issues, detection and management strategies. Toxins (Basel). 2023;15(4):246. https://doi.org/10.3390/toxins15040246. PMID: 37104184; PMCID: PMC10140874.
9. Liu ZM, Li LQ, Peng MH, et al. Hepatitis B virus infection contributes to oxidative stress in a population exposed to aflatoxin B1 and high-risk for hepatocellular carcinoma. Cancer Lett. 2008;263:212–22.
10. Omer RE, Verhoef L, Van't Veer P, et al. Peanut butter intake, GSTM1 genotype and hepatocellular carcinoma: a case-control study in Sudan. Cancer Causes Control. 2001;12:23–32.
11. Martins C, Vidal A, De Boevre M, DeSaeger S, Nunes C, Torres D, Goios A, Lopes C, Alvito P, Assunção R. Burden of disease associated with dietary exposure to carcinogenic aflatoxins in Portugal using human biomonitoring approach. Food Res Int. 2020;134:109210.
12. Groopman JD, Croy RG, Wogan GN. In vitro reactions of aflatoxin B1-adducted DNA. Proc Natl Acad Sci USA. 1981;78:5445–9.
13. Nayak S, Sashidhar RB, Bhat RV. Quantification and validation of enzyme immunoassay for urinary aflatoxin B_1–N^7-guanine adduct for biological monitoring of aflatoxins. Analyst. 2001;126:179–83.

8.1 Overview

8.1.1 Exposure of the General Population

In the general population, the causes of exposure to 4-aminobiphenyl are cigarette smoking and passive inhalation of tobacco [1]. 4-Aminobiphenyl can occur as a contaminant in 2-aminobiphenyl, which is used in the manufacture of dyes. Other potential sources include aniline, drugs, cosmetics, color additives in food, clothes, and hair dyes [1–3]. 4-Aminobiphenyl has also been found as a contaminant in diphenylamine, a fungicide used on apples, as well as in cooking oil fumes. In a study from Taiwan (China), concentrations of 4-aminobiphenyl were 35.7 $\mu g/m^3$ in sunflower oil cooking fumes, 26.4 $\mu g/m3$ in vegetable oil fumes, and 23.3 $\mu g/m^3$ in refined lard oil fat [4]. Living near places contaminated with benzidine can lead to exposure, as certain bacteria can degrade benzidine in the environment to 4-aminobiphenyl [5]. There are likely other sources of environmental exposure, as biomarkers derived from aromatic amines, such as hemoglobin adducts or metabolites in urine, have also been identified in nonsmokers not occupationally exposed to these chemicals [1, 6].

4-Aminobiphenyl causes bladder cancer and is carcinogenic to humans [1]. Its urinary metabolites are N-hydroxy-4-aminobiphenyl, N-glucuronides, and 4-aminobiphenyl-DNA adducts [6].

V. Radosavljevic, *Assessing Human Exposure to Key Chemical Carcinogens*, https://doi.org/10.1007/978-3-031-84441-6_8

Appendix: Exposure Evaluation Questionnaire

1. During the last few days, have you smoked or been exposed to tobacco smoke and to what extent? ....
....
....

2. During the last few days, were you exposed to oil fumes during frying for several hours and to what extent? ....
....
....

3. During the last few days, have you been exposed to aniline dyes or dyes in general and to what extent? ....
....
....

4. During the last few days, have you been exposed to hair dyes and to what extent?
....
....
....

5. During the last few days, have you sprayed apples or other fruits against fungi and to what extent? ....
....
....

6. Do you consume food containing colors and how often: ....
....
....
....
   (a) Daily
   (b) Three times a week
   (c) Once a week or less often

7. Do you use cosmetic products that contain colors and how often: ....
....
....
....
   (a) Daily
   (b) Three times a week
   (c) Once a week or less often

8. Do you use colored laundry and how often: ....
....
....
....
   (a) Daily
   (b) Three times a week
   (c) Once a week or less often

References

1. IARC. Some aromatic amines, organic dyes, and related exposures. IARC Monogr Eval Carcinog Risks Hum. 2010;99:1–678.
2. Souza MCO, González N, Herrero M, Marquès M, Rovira J, Nadal M, et al. Screening of regulated aromatic amines in clothing marketed in Brazil and Spain: assessment of human health risks. Environ Res. 2023;221:115264. https://doi.org/10.1016/j.envres.2023.115264.
3. More SL, Fung ES, Mathis C, Schulte AM, Hollins D. Dermal exposure and hair dye: assessing potential bladder cancer risk from permanent hair dye. Regul Toxicol Pharmacol. 2023;138:105331. https://doi.org/10.1016/j.yrtph.2022.105331.
4. Chiang T-A, Pei-Fen W, Ying LS, et al. Mutagenicity and aromatic amine content of fumes from heated cooking oils produced in Taiwan. Food Chem Toxicol. 1999;37:125–34.
5. Bafana A, Devi SS, Krishnamurthi K, Chakrabarti T. Kinetics of decolourisation and biotransformation of direct black 38 by C. Hominis and P. Stutzeri. Appl Microbiol Biotechnol. 2007;74:1145–52.
6. Radosavljevic V. Urinary markers/metabolites of exposure to chemical carcinogens—new possibilities in preventive oncology. Ecotoxicol Environ Saf. 2024;269:115774.

9.1 Overview

9.1.1 Occurrence in the Environment and Traditional Use

Aristolochia species are ubiquitous and have been used (*A. contorta, A. debilis, A. fangchi,* and *A. manshuriensis*) in traditional Chinese medicine as antirheumatic and diuretic and in the treatment of edema. Their medicinal use in traditional Indian medicine is very limited. Some authors have reported [1] that aristolochic acid occurring in *Aristolochia species* used in traditional herbal medicines has the function of phospholipase A2 inhibitor and as an antineoplastic, antiseptic, anti-inflammatory, and bactericidal agent. A*ristolochia acids (AAs)* are found in the *Aristolochiaceae* family, which includes about 500 species, spread all around the world, with most of the taxa in the tropical region and are widely used as herbal remedies [2]. Urothelial cancer development requires at least several years of constant exposure to the levels of AAs usually found in *Aristolochia*-based herbal remedies [2]. The occurrence of *AAs* in either the above- or underground parts of vegetables is attributed to a specific passage route that could explain how AAs are transported within the environment. Some results show that AAs' presence is attributed to the growing of *A. clematitis* in the area, and in general, the highest concentrations are found in the soil samples, and the lowest concentrations in cucumber and fruit, but without a direct correlation to the distance (or 50 cm) from the *Aristolochia* plants [3]. In the 1990s, their use for weight loss in developed countries was prohibited or strictly limited. Since then, *AAs* have been produced commercially only as a reference standard and as research chemicals [4].

Aristolochic acid adducts and DNA were found in urothelial tissue samples from all urothelial cancer patients with Chinese herbal nephropathy [5]. Their urinary metabolites are aristolactam I (a metabolite of aristolochic acid I) and aristolactam II (a metabolite of aristolochic acid II). Apart from aristolactam, DNA adducts are also their urinary metabolites [6].

V. Radosavljevic, *Assessing Human Exposure to Key Chemical Carcinogens*,
https://doi.org/10.1007/978-3-031-84441-6_9

Appendix: Exposure Evaluation Questionnaire

1. Have you used slimming products?   (a) Yes   (b) No
2. If you used slimming products, which ones and for how long? ....
   ....
   ....
3. In the last week, have you consumed bulb vegetables, cucumber, or lettuce every day (which ones and for how long)?...
   ....
   ....
4. Do you suffer from chronic kidney failure and/or urinary tract cancer? ....
   ....
5. Are there people in your area suffering from chronic kidney failure and/or urinary tract cancer and in what number? ....
   ....
   ....
6. Do you live in an area known for suffering from Balkan endemic nephropathy (how long)?...
   ....

References

1. Buckingham J, editor. Dictionary of natural products on CD-ROM. Boca Raton: CRC Press/ Chapman & Hall/CRC; 2001.
2. Lukinich-Gruia AT, Nortier J, Pavlovic NM, Milovanovic D, Popovic M, Draghia LP, Paunescu V, Tatu CA. Aristolochic acid I as an emerging biogenic contaminant involved in chronic kidney diseases: a comprehensive review on exposure pathways, environmental health issues and future challenges. Chemosphere. 2022;297:134111.
3. Draghia LP, Lukinich-Gruia AT, Oprean C, Pavlovic NM, Paunescu V, Tatu CA. Aristolochic acid I: an investigation into the role of food crops contamination, as a potential natural exposure pathway. Environ Geochem Health. 2021; https://doi.org/10.1007/s10653-021-009034.
4. Sigma-Aldrich. Biochemicals and reagents for life science research 2002–2003. St. Louis: Sigma; 2002. p. 220.
5. Radosavljević V. Urinary markers of exposure to chemical carcinogens—new guidelines in preventive oncology. Belgrade: Media Center "Defense"; 2024. (in Serbian).
6. Radosavljevic V. Urinary markers/metabolites of exposure to chemical carcinogens—new possibilities in preventive oncology. Ecotoxicol Environ Saf. 2024;269:115774.

Human Exposure to Benzene 10

10.1 Overview

10.1.1 Exposure of the General Population

Exposure to benzene is highest in industrial areas, followed by motor vehicle exhaust and fuel vapor from gas stations [1, 2]. For example, for a 1-h exposure, the intake of benzene while driving a motor vehicle is estimated to be 40 μg. Exposure is greater for people who spend significant time in motor vehicles in congested traffic areas [3, 4]. The primary sources of benzene exposure for the general population are ambient air containing tobacco smoke, air in heavy traffic areas, gas station environments, contaminated water, and contaminated food [5]. In the general population of the United Kingdom, it has been estimated that infants (<1 year), children up to 11 years of age and nonoccupationally exposed adults receive average daily doses of benzene ranging from 15 to 26 μg, 29 to 50 μg, and 75 to 522 μg, respectively [6].

Benzene is mostly used in the production of organic chemicals such as styrene, polystyrene, various styrene copolymers, latexes and resins, phenol, cyclohexane, aniline, alkylbenzenes (used in detergents), and chlorobenzenes [7]. Also, benzene is an intermediate in the production of anthraquinone, hydroquinone, benzene hexachloride, cyclohexane, benzene sulfonic acid, and other products used in drugs, dyes, insecticides, nylon monomers, and plastics [8]. Benzene occurs naturally in crude oil and gasoline and is added to unleaded gasoline for its ability to increase octane and anti-knock. The concentration of benzene in these fuels is typically 1–2% by volume [4]. Therefore, employees in workplaces exposed to exhaust gases from motor vehicles are highly exposed to benzene [4]. In the USA, potential exposure to benzene occurred in agriculture, during oil and gas extraction, construction, production of food products, tobacco, textiles, lumber and wood, printing and publishing, exposure to oil and coal products, rubber production, leather production, and transport and health services [9]. In the People's Republic of China industries

© The Author(s), under exclusive license to Springer Nature Switzerland AG 2025

V. Radosavljevic, *Assessing Human Exposure to Key Chemical Carcinogens*, https://doi.org/10.1007/978-3-031-84441-6_10

with the highest reported exposure are leather, electronic devices, machinery, footwear, office supplies, and sports equipment [10].

Benzene causes acute myeloid leukemia/acute nonlymphocytic leukemia, and positive associations between benzene exposure and acute lymphocytic leukemia, chronic lymphocytic leukemia, multiple myeloma, and non-Hodgkin's leukemia have been observed [11]. Urinary trans, trans-muconic acid (t,t-MA), and S-phenylmercapturic acid (S-FMA) are sensitive markers for recent low-level benzene exposure [12].

Appendix: Exposure Evaluation Questionnaire

1. During the last week, were you exposed to fire and for how long?..................
   ....
   ....

2. Are you employed and in what jobs in:
   - Oil, natural gas, or refineries industry
   - Chemical industry (specify what type of chemical industry, pay particular attention to the styrene or Styrofoam industry)...................................
     ....
   - Footwear industry
   - Rubber industry
   - Printers

3. During the last week, have you been exposed to:
   - Colors
   - Varnishes
   - Nail polish remover
   - Industrial solvents
   - Gasoline and other fuels
   - Glues
   - Furniture wax
   - Detergents
   - Adhesives and coatings
   - Tires
   - Crude oil
   - Means for industrial cleaning and degreasing
   - Exhaust gases of motor vehicles (at least 1 h a day)

4. During the last week, have you been near landfills and/or gas stations and for how long? ....
   ....
   ....

5. Are you a smoker or have you been exposed to tobacco smoke in the last few days?..............
   ....
   ....

6. Have you consumed smoked or canned fish in the last few days and in what quantity? ....

7. Have you consumed greasy salads (Russian, French, chicken, tzatziki, etc.) in recent days and in what quantity?...

....

....

....

8. Have you consumed smoked, cured meat, fermented, and/or preserved meat in the last days and in what quantity?...

....

....

....

9. Have you consumed the following spices, vanilla, mint, orange concentrate, hazelnuts, chocolate, pistachios, cola, and concentrated fruit juices, in the last few days? Which and in which faces?...

....

....

....

10. Have you consumed food in the last few days to which benzoates, benzoic acid, vitamin C, and acidity regulators have been added, and in what quantity?

....

....

....

References

1. Boogaard PJ. Human biomonitoring of lowlevel benzene exposures. Crit Rev Toxicol. 2022;52(10):799–810. https://doi.org/10.1080/10408444.2023.2175642.
2. Loomis D, Guyton KZ, Grosse Y, El Ghissassi F, Bouvard V, Benbrahim-Tallaa L, Guha N, Vilahur N, Mattock H, Straif K, International Agency for Research on Cancer Monograph Working Group. Carcinogenicity of benzene. Lancet Oncol. 2017;18:1574–5. https://doi.org/10.1016/S1470-2045(17)30832-X.
3. NTP. Benzene. NTP 11th report on carcinogens. Rep Carcinog. 2005;11:1–A32.
4. ATSDR. Toxicological profile for benzene. Atlanta: Agency for Toxic Substances and Disease Registry; 2007. p. 438.
5. Vinci RM, Jacxsens L, Van Loco J, Matsiko E, Lachat C, de Schaetzen T, Canfyn M, Van Overmeire I, Kolsteren P, De Meulenaer B. Assessment of human exposure to benzene through foods from the Belgian market. Chemosphere. 2012;88:1001–7.
6. Duarte-Davidson R, Courage C, Rushton L, Levy L. Benzene in the environment: an assessment of the potential risks to the health of the population. Occup Environ Med. 2001;58:2–13.
7. Kirschner M. Chemical profile: benzene. ICIS Chemical Business; 2009. Available at http://www.icis.com/Articles/2009/02/16/9192064/Chemical-profileBenzene.html
8. Burridge E. Chemical profile: benzene. ICIS Chem Bus (Europe/Middle East/Asia). 2007;2(57):36.
9. NIOSH. National Occupational Exposure Survey (1981–83). Cincinnati: US Department of Health and Human Services, Public Health Service, National Institute for Occupational Safety and Health; 1990. http://www.cdc.gov/noes/noes2/09070occ.html

10. Liang Y-X, Wong O, Armstrong T, et al. An overview of published benzene exposure data by industry in China, 1960-2003. Chem Biol Interact. 2005;153-154:55–64.
11. Radosavljević V. Urinary markers of exposure to chemical carcinogens—new guidelines in preventive oncology. Belgrade: Media Center "Defense"; 2024. (in Serbian).
12. Radosavljevic V. Urinary markers/metabolites of exposure to chemical carcinogens—new possibilities in preventive oncology. Ecotoxicol Environ Saf. 2024;269:115774.

Human Exposure to Benzidine

11

11.1 Overview

11.1.1 Exposure of the General Population

The general population may be exposed to benzidine through contact with leather products [1], clothing, and toys [2] containing benzidine or benzidine-based paints [3–5]. The food dyes tartrazine and sunset yellow contain trace amounts of benzidine (within nanograms per gram of food) [6].

The production and use of benzidine in the production of paints has been recorded in some developing countries (the transfer of benzidine production from other European countries to the former Serbia and Montenegro and the Republic of Korea) [7–9]. Exposure to benzidine through ingestion is unlikely, but other impurities in synthetic dyes may be metabolized to benzidine after ingestion [10].

Benzidine causes bladder cancer [11]. Its urinary metabolites are benzidine and benzidine conjugates (monoacetylbenzidine) [12].

Appendix: Exposure Evaluation Questionnaire

1. Have you been in contact with colors, in particular azo dyes? When, how, and how long? ....
   ....

2. Have you been in contact with colored leather or textiles, esp. azo dyes? When, in what way, and for how long? ....
   ....
   ....

3. Have you been in contact with paper dyes or colored paper (esp azo dyes)? When, in what way, and for how long? ....

© The Author(s), under exclusive license to Springer Nature
Switzerland AG 2025
V. Radosavljevic, *Assessing Human Exposure to Key Chemical Carcinogens*,
https://doi.org/10.1007/978-3-031-84441-6_11

4. Have you been in contact with colored toys, esp. azo dyes? When, in what way, and for how long? ....

5. Did you live near paint factories, especially azo dye? When, in what way, and for how long? ....

References

1. Ahlström LH, Sparr Eskilsson C, Björklund E. Determination of banned azo dyes in consumer goods. Trends Anal Chem. 2005;24:49–56.
2. Garrigós MC, Reche F, Marín ML, Jiménez A. Determination of aromatic amines formed from azo colorants in toy products. J Chromatogr A. 2002;976:309–17.
3. National Cancer Institute USA. 2024. https://www.cancer.gov/about-cancer/causes-prevention/risk/substances/benzidine. Accessed 18 Sept 2024.
4. Agency for Toxic Substances and Disease Registry (ATSDR). Toxicological profile for benzidine. Atlanta: U.S. Public Health Service, U.S. Department of Health and Human Services; 1995.
5. California Environmental Protection Agency (CalEPA). Technical support document for the determination of noncancer chronic reference exposure levels. Berkeley: Draft for Public Comment. Office of Environmental Health Hazard Assessment; 1997.
6. Lancaster FE, Lawrence JF. Determination of benzidine in the food colours tartrazine and sunset yellow FCF, by reduction and derivatization followed by high-performance liquid chromatography [abstract]. Food Addit Contam. 1999;16:381–90.
7. Carreón T, Le Masters GK, Ruder AM, Schulte PA. The genetic and environmental factors involved in benzidine metabolism and bladder carcinogenesis in exposed workers. Front Biosci. 2006;11:2889–902.
8. U.S. Department of Health and Human Services. Hazardous Substances Data Bank (HSDB, online database). Bethesda: National Toxicology Information Program, National Library of Medicine; 1993.
9. U.S. Environmental Protection Agency. Integrated Risk Information System (IRIS) on benzidine. Washington, DC: National Center for Environmental Assessment, Office of Research and Development; 1999.
10. ATSDR. Toxicological profile for benzidine. Atlanta: Agency for Toxic Substances and Disease Registry; 2001. p. 242.
11. Radosavljević V. Urinarni markeri ekspozicije hemijskim kancerogenima—nove smernice u preventivnoj onkologiji (Urinary markers of exposure to chemical carcinogens—new guidelines in preventive oncology). Beograd: Medija centar „Odbrana"; 2024.
12. Radosavljevic V. Urinary markers/metabolites of exposure to chemical carcinogens—new possibilities in preventive oncology. Ecotoxicol Environ Saf. 2024; https://doi.org/10.1016/j.ecoenv.2023.115774.

12.1 Overview

Benzo[a]pyrene belongs to the group of polycyclic aromatic hydrocarbons (PAHs), highly carcinogenic compounds [1]. They are ubiquitous environmental pollutants (in air, water, soil, and sediments), mostly in trace amounts, except near their sources [2, 3]. PAHs are formed during incomplete combustion or pyrolysis of organic material [4]. Tobacco and tobacco smoke contain high concentrations of PAHs [5]. Moreover, PAHs are present in some foods and in several pharmaceutical products [5].

12.1.1 Exposure of the General Population

The general population can be exposed to benzo[a]pyrene through tobacco smoke, air, water, soil, food, and pharmaceutical products [2]. Benzo[a]pyrene concentrations in sidestream cigarette smoke range from 52 to 95 ng per cigarette [6]. Other major sources of benzo[a]pyrene are wood and coal heating [4, 7]. Much smaller amounts of benzo[a]pyrene are produced by oil and gas heating, cooking, exhaust gases from motor vehicles (especially diesel engines), industrial emissions, and forest fires [4]. However, very high concentrations have been recorded in road tunnels and large cities that heavily use coal or other biomass as heating fuel [2, 8]. Estimates of dietary intake of benzo[a]pyrene are a maximum of several micrograms per person per day. Dietary sources of PAHs include roasted, grilled, and smoked meats, as well as fruits and vegetables grown on contaminated soil (usually areas with surface contamination of atmospheric benzo[a]pyrene) [5].

Exposure to benzo[a]pyrene is associated with cancers of the lung, bladder, skin, esophagus, hematolymphatic system, lips, oral cavity, and pharynx [6, 9].

Its urinary metabolites are benzo[a]pyrene-r-7, t-8, t-9, c-10-tetrahydrotetrol, BPT I-1, and benzo[a]pyrene-r-7, t-8, c-9, c-10-tetrahydrotetrol, BPT II-1 [10].

V. Radosavljevic, *Assessing Human Exposure to Key Chemical Carcinogens*,
https://doi.org/10.1007/978-3-031-84441-6_12

Appendix: Exposure Evaluation Questionnaire

1. Are you exposed to burning wood or coal? When, how often, and in what situation-pit?..
   ....

2. Are you exposed to machine oil? When, how often, and in what situations?..........
   ....
   ....

3. Do you work or live near thermal power plants or coal mines?

4. Do you work or live near a factory and what kind? ....

5. Do you work or live near a landfill and what kind? ....

6. Are you exposed to exhaust gases from motor vehicles? In what way and how much time a day?..
   ....

7. Are you exposed to biomass burning? In what way and how much time a day?.
   ....
   ....

8. Do you work or live near a metal industry and what kind?..............................
   ....
   ....

9. Do you work or live in a rural or urban environment? ....
   ....
   ....

10. Do you live or work in blocks of buildings along boulevards or important roads?
    ....
    ....
    ....
    ....

11. Do you live or work near large parking lots or intersections?
    ....
    ....

12. Do you live or work near railway (tram) stations or near traffic tra cks?..
    ....
    ....
    ....

13. Do you have a garden next to roads (roads or railways) or streets?.............
    ....
    ....

14. Are there people in your neighborhood or colleagues at work suffering from lung, skin, or bladder cancer?..
    ....

15. Have there been any cases of premature or mentally handicapped children in your   neighborhood?..
....

16. Do you use water from rivers and/or lakes that are in the immediate vicinity of landfills, metal industries, thermal power plants, coal mines, refineries, or chemical industries?
....
....

17. In the last week, have you consumed oils, fats, smoked fish and/or meat, sweets, or other highly processed cereal products? If so, specify which ones, when, and how much?

18. Were you exposed to tobacco smoke during the previous 5 days and to what extent?
....
....

19. Do you work in the construction of roads and sidewalks (especially during the last 10 days)?......
....
....

20. Do you work as a truck, bus driver or have you had long drives in motor vehicles in the last week? ....
....
....

21. Are you a traffic driver or a chimney sweep, or do you work in the coal industry or in wood impregnation? ....
....

22. Did you consume grilled meat, spring barley during the last week, or drinks made from wild barley (when and in what quantity)?...
....
....
....

References

1. Ziling Y, Xiang M, Ma R, Yi C, Guocheng H, Chen X, Liu Y, Yunjiang Y. Development of human health criteria in China for benzo[a]pyrene: a comparison of deterministic and probabilistic approaches. Chemosphere. 2023;320:138104.
2. Bukowska B, Mokra K, Michałowicz J. Benzo[a]pyrene—environmental occurrence, human exposure, and mechanisms of toxicity. Int J Mol Sci. 2022;23:6348. https://doi.org/10.3390/ijms23116348.
3. Liao K, Jian Zhen Y. Abundance and sources of benzo[a]pyrene and other PAHs in ambient air in Hong Kong: a review of 20-year measurements (1997e2016). Chemosphere. 2020;259:127518.
4. Guerreiro CBB, Horalek J, de Leeuw F, Couvidat F. Benzo(a)pyrene in Europe: ambient air concentrations, population exposure and health effects. Environ Pollut. 2016;214:657e667.

5. IARC. Some non-heterocyclic polycyclic aromatic hydrocarbons and some related exposures. IARC Monogr Eval Carcinog Risks Hum. 2010;92:1–853.
6. Radosavljević V. Urinarni markeri ekspozicije hemijskim kancerogenima—nove smernice u preventivnoj onkologiji (Urinary markers of exposure to chemical carcinogens—new guidelines in preventive oncology). Beograd: Medija centar „Odbrana"; 2024.
7. Boente C, Baragano D, Gallego JR. Benzo[a]pyrene sourcing and abundance in a coal region in transition reveals historical pollution, rendering soil screening levels impractical. Environ Pollut. 2020;266:115341.
8. Kosheleva NE, Vlasov DV, Timofeev IV, Samsonov TE, Kasimov NS. Benzo[a]pyrene in Moscow road dust: pollution levels and health risks. Environ Geochem Health. 2023;45:1669–94. https://doi.org/10.1007/s10653-022-01287-9.
9. Xue W, Warshawsky D. Metabolic activation of polycyclic and heterocyclic aromatic hydrocarbons and DNA damage: a review. Toxicol Appl Pharmacol. 2005;206:73–93.
10. Radosavljevic V. Urinary markers/metabolites of exposure to chemical carcinogens—new possibilities in preventive oncology. Ecotoxicol Environ Saf. 2024;269:115774.

Human Exposure to Bis(Chloromethyl)Ether (BHME) and Chloromethyl Methyl Ether (HMME)

13.1 Overview

BHME and HMME are primarily used as chemical intermediates and alkylating agents. BHME is used as a laboratory reagent in the production of plastics, ion exchange resins and polymers [1]. Uses of BHME include the cross-linking of cellulose, the preparation of styrene and other polymers, the surface treatment of vulcanized rubber to increase adhesion, and the production of flame-resistant fabrics [2]. HMME is used as an alkylating agent and industrial solvent for the production of dodecylbenzyl chloride, water repellents, ion exchange resins and polymers, and a chloromethylation reagent [1]. The most likely source of exposure to BHME is during the production or use of chemicals, where it may be present as a contaminant or formed unintentionally [1].

13.1.1 Exposure of the General Population

The primary routes of potential human exposure to technical grade BHME and HMME are inhalation and dermal contact. Almost all releases of BHME and HMME to the environment were aerogenic [3].

Bis(chloromethyl)ether and chloromethyl methyl ether (technical grade) cause lung cancer. BHME and HMME are subject to rapid hydrolysis to formaldehyde and hydrochloric acid. A specific, persistent, and reliable urinary metabolite is not known [4].

© The Author(s), under exclusive license to Springer Nature
Switzerland AG 2025
V. Radosavljevic, *Assessing Human Exposure to Key Chemical Carcinogens*,
https://doi.org/10.1007/978-3-031-84441-6_13

Appendix: Exposure Evaluation Questionnaire

1. Do you work in a chemical laboratory and in what jobs?..................................
....
....

2. Do you work in the textile industry and in what jobs?..................................
....
....

3. Do you work in the pulp and/or Styrofoam industry and in what jobs?................
....
....

4. Do you work in the rubber industry and in what jobs?..................................
....
....

5. Do you work in the resin and polymer industry and in what jobs?.......................
....
....

6. Do you work in the industry of plastics and/or waterproof materials and in which
   position?
   Hunting?..
....

7. Do you work in the chlorine industry and in what jobs?..................................
....

References

1. HSDB. Hazardous Substances Data Bank. Bethesda: National Library of Medicine; 2003. http://toxnet.nlm.nih.gov/cgi-bin/sis/htmlgen?HSDB
2. IARC. Chemical agents and related occupations. IARC Monogr Eval Carcinog Risks Hum. 2012;100F:1–628.
3. US EPA. United States Environmental Protection Agency. Toxics Release Inventory program (TRI). 2003.
4. Radosavljević V. Urinarni markeri ekspozicije hemijskim kancerogenima—nove smernice u preventivnoj onkologiji (Urinary markers of exposure to chemical carcinogens—new guidelines in preventive oncology). Beograd: Medija centar „Odbrana"; 2024.

14.1 Overview

14.1.1 Occurrence in the Environment

1,3-Butadiene is not known as a natural product. It is a ubiquitous environmental pollutant and mainly originates from combustion products (motor vehicle emissions, tobacco smoke) [1, 2]. It is a colorless gas and more than 95% of the world's production is a co-product of the industrial synthesis of ethylene [3]. It is estimated that 9.3 million tons of 1,3-butadiene were produced in the world in 2005 [4]. Asia is now its largest producer. Vehicles with an emission control device (catalyst) had an average emission rate of 2.1 ± 1.5 mg/km [5]. Based on an average of 20,000 km per year per car and roughly over a billion registered cars in the world and taking into account estimated average emission rates [5], butadiene emissions from car exhaust can be estimated at around tens of millions of tons per year [4]. Butadiene is also released into the atmosphere from smoke from fires, burning plastics, and evaporation from petrol [6, 7]. In the United Kingdom in 1996, the estimated emission of butadiene in road vehicle exhaust was 68%, and emissions from machinery were 14%. The remaining emissions came from the chemical industry [1]. Products containing butadiene are incorporated into automotive components, building materials, appliance parts, computers and telecommunications equipment, clothing, protective clothing, packaging, and household items [8]. Butadiene is also used as an intermediate in the production of chloroprene, adiponitrile, and other basic petrochemicals [8].

The strongest evidence exists for an association with non-Hodgkin's lymphoma (study of workers in the monomer industry) [9]. The following urinary metabolites were identified: 1,2-dihydroxybutyl mercapturic acid (DHBMA) and monohydroxy-3-butenyl mercapturic acid (MHBMA) [10].

57

V. Radosavljevic, *Assessing Human Exposure to Key Chemical Carcinogens*, https://doi.org/10.1007/978-3-031-84441-6_14

Appendix: Exposure Evaluation Questionnaire

1. Are you a tobacco user? ....
2. Do you work or live near an oil refinery? ....
3. Do you work or live near the synthetic materials industry, especially synthetic rubber and thermoplastic resins? ....
4. Do you work or live near a landfill for synthetic materials? ....
5. Do you work or live near major roads? ....
6. Are you exposed to exhaust gases from motor vehicles and for how long? ....
7. Do you work in the oil and gas extraction industry or do you live near an oil and gas extraction facility? ....
8. Are you exposed to stubble burning or other burnings in agriculture and how much?...
9. Are you exposed to forest fires or the burning of bushes or other vegetation and how much?...
10. Do you work or live near a landfill? ....
11. Were you exposed to burning biomass (wood, leaves, twigs, straw), when, and for how long? ....
12. Do you work or live near a plant where oil is heated at high temperatures? ....
13. Do you work or live near a plant where paper or cardboard is produced? ....
14. Are you often exposed to electrosurgical procedures and how much? ....
15. Do you work or live near a coal mine?...
16. Do you work as a hairdresser? ....

References

1. Chen W-Q, Zhang X-Y. 1,3-butadiene: a ubiquitous environmental mutagen and its associations with diseases. Gene Environ. 2022;44:3. https://doi.org/10.1186/s41021-021-00233-y.
2. Australian Government. Department of Climate Change, Energy, the Environment and Water. 2022. https://www.dcceew.gov.au/environment/protection/npi/substances/fact-sheets/13-butadiene-vinyl-ethylene. Accessed 17 Sept 2024.
3. IARC. 1,3-Butadiene, ethylene oxide and vinyl halides (vinyl fluoride, vinyl chloride and vinyl bromide). IARC monographs on the evaluation of carcinogenic risks to humans, 97, Lyon, 2008. p. 45–184.
4. CMAI (Chemical Marketing Associates International). Product focus. Butadiene. Chem Week, 2006, February 8. p. 26.
5. Ye Y, Galbally IE, Weeks IA. Emission of 1,3-butadiene from petrol-driven motor vehicle. Atmos Environ. 1997;31:1157–65.
6. Agency for Toxic Substances and Disease Registry. Toxicological profile for 1,3-butadiene (Report No. TR-91/07), 1992, Atlanta, GA.
7. IARC. Occupational exposures to mists and vapours from strong inorganic acids; and other industrial chemicals. IARC monographs on the evaluation of carcinogenic risks to humans, vol. 54, Lyon, 1992. p. 237–285.
8. White WC. Butadiene production process overview. Chem Biol Interact. 2007;166:10–4.
9. Radosavljević V. Urinarni markeri ekspozicije hemijskim kancerogenima—nove smernice u preventivnoj onkologiji (Urinary markers of exposure to chemical carcinogens—new guidelines in preventive oncology). Beograd: Medija centar „Odbrana"; 2024.
10. Radosavljevic V. Urinary markers/metabolites of exposure to chemical carcinogens—new possibilities in preventive oncology. Ecotoxicol Environ Saf. 2024; https://doi.org/10.1016/j.ecoenv.2023.115774.

15.1 Overview

Atmospheric air samples from rural and urban areas usually do not contain detectable levels of vinyl chloride (VC) [1]. Vinyl chloride is released into the environment from the plastics industry—emissions to the atmosphere or wastewater in surface waters [2]. Also, it is released as a product of decomposition of chlorinated solvents in landfills as landfill gas. VC is released from landfills into groundwater [3]. People living near the plastics industry are likely exposed to high concentrations of vinyl chloride in the air, and their average daily intake could be as high as several milligrams [1, 2].

Over 95% of vinyl chloride monomer (VCM) is used to produce its polymer—polyvinyl chloride (PVC). Vinyl chloride is used to a lesser extent in the production of chlorinated solvents and the production of ethylene diamine for the production of resins [2–4]. PVC makes up a significant percentage of the total use of plastics worldwide [3]. The largest use of PVC is in the production of plastic piping, floor coverings, consumer goods, electrical applications, and transportation.

The general population can be exposed to VCM/PVC through inhalation of contaminated air, ingestion of contaminated drinking water, consumption of contaminated food, and dermal contact [2]. Fortunately, exposure levels for most of the population are very low [1]. Residues in PVC resin and PVC products may contain VCM that is released into the environment. Also, in daily life, VCM is released from plastic bottles, toys, kitchen utensils, food wrappers, wallpaper, pipes, car interiors, bathroom tiles, and cigarettes (14–27 ng/cigarette) [5]. Exposure to vinyl chloride in drinking water for most of the population is unlikely, and the US Environmental Protection Agency has estimated that approximately 0.9% of the US population is exposed to vinyl chloride in drinking water at concentrations of 1.0 µg/l or higher, while 0.3% is exposed to concentrations higher than 5 µg/l [1].

Vinyl chloride causes liver angiosarcoma and hepatocellular carcinoma [6]. Its urinary metabolites are vinyl chloride and thiodiglycolic acid [7].

V. Radosavljevic, *Assessing Human Exposure to Key Chemical Carcinogens*, https://doi.org/10.1007/978-3-031-84441-6_15

Appendix: Exposure Evaluation Questionnaire

1. Do you work or live near plastic factories or landfills? ....
   ....

2. Do you work or live near the oil shale industry? ....
   ....

3. Do you work or live near plastic resin factories? ....
   ....

4. Do you work or live near factories that use plastic in any way? ....
   ....
   ....

5. Are you in any intensive contact with plastic products (food packaging, toys, household appliances, etc.)? ....
   ....
   ....
   ....

References

1. NTP. Vinyl chloride report on carcinogens, eleventh edition. Rep Carcinog. 2005;11:1–A32.
2. U.S. Department of Health and Human Services. Agency for Toxic Substances and Disease Registry. Toxicological profile for vinyl chloride. 2024, January.
3. WHO. Vinyl chloride, Environmental health criteria 215. Geneva: World Health Organization; 1999.
4. European Commission. Integrated Pollution Prevention and Control (IPPC). Luxembourg: Reference Document on Best Available Techniques in the Large Volume Organic Chemical Industry; 2003.
5. IARC. Tobacco smoke and involuntary smoking. IARC Monogr Eval Carcinog Risks Hum. 2004;83:1–1438.
6. Radosavljević V. Urinarni markeri ekspozicije hemijskim kancerogenima—nove smernice u preventivnoj onkologiji (Urinary markers of exposure to chemical carcinogens—new guidelines in preventive oncology). Beograd: Medija centar „Odbrana"; 2024.
7. Radosavljevic V. Urinary markers/metabolites of exposure to chemical carcinogens—new possibilities in preventive oncology. Ecotoxicol Environ Saf. 2024; https://doi.org/10.1016/j.ecoenv.2023.115774.

Human Exposure to 1,2-Dichloropropane

16

16.1 Overview

2-Dichloropropane is not known to occur in nature.

1,2-Dichloropropane is primarily used as a chemical intermediate in the production of other organic chemicals, such as propylene, carbon tetrachloride, and tetrachloroethylene [1]. It is also used in textile stain removers, oil and paraffin extractors, scouring compounds, metal cleaners [1, 2], degreasers and solvent-based cleaning products, paint removers, and adhesives [1, 3] and is an ingredient in insecticides. It was formerly used as one component of a grain and soil fumigant, although such use is no longer permitted in Europe and the US [4].

Commercial 1,2-dichloropropane is sold as a high-purity liquid (purity 99–99.5%) for industrial use. It was produced in North and South America, Europe, and Asia. The total annual world production of 1,2-dichloropropane for 2001 was estimated at 350,000 tons. In 2003, the estimated percentage of regional production of 1,2-dichloropropane was 64–69% in North America, 19–25% in Europe, 9–10% in South America, and 2–3% in Japan [5]. Production in the USA declined in the early 1980s, as it was no longer used for paint stripping, furniture finishing, or as an insecticide [2, 6, 7]. The amount produced and imported into European Union countries was between 1000 and 10,000 tons per year [3]. Annual production of 1,2-dichloropropane in China is estimated at 45,000–68,000 tons [8]. In Japan, in 2011, the reported annual production and import was 1400 tons [9]. Very little information was available on the exposure of the general population to 1,2-dichloropropane. Exposure can occur through inhalation of contaminated air or ingestion of contaminated water.

There is sufficient evidence of the carcinogenicity of 1,2-dichloropropane, which causes cancer of the biliary tract (cholangiocarcinoma) in humans [10]. Its urinary metabolite is 1,2-dichloropropane [11].

V. Radosavljevic, *Assessing Human Exposure to Key Chemical Carcinogens*, https://doi.org/10.1007/978-3-031-84441-6_16

Appendix: Exposure Evaluation Questionnaire

1. Are you in any contact with industrial waxes or preparations containing them? Specify which preparations, type, and time of contact...

2. Are you in any contact with chemical sealants or preparations containing them? Specify which preparations, type, and time of contact...

3. Do you work or live near chlorinated solvents, plastics, lubricants and oils, or rubber industries? Specify the type of industry, type, and time of exposure..

4. Are you in any contact with stain removers, paraffin removers, cleaning or degreasing agents, galvanizers, or preparations containing them? Specify which preparations, type, and time of contact...

5. Do you work or live near a place where waste is incinerated? Specify the type of incinerator, type, and time of exposure...

6. Do you work or live near a place where there is intensive burning of motor fuels? Specify the type, and time of exposure...

7. Do you work or live near the place where there is a gas station? Specify the type and time of exposure...

8. Have you been exposed to fumigants? Specify the type and time of exposure..

   ....

9. Have you been exposed to paint removers, varnishes, or means for removing the finish of furniture? Specify the type and time of exposure...

   ....

10. Have you been exposed to the industry of chemical and related products, machines (except electrical), finished metal products, textile products, or photographic film? Specify the type and time of exposure..

    ....

11. Do you work or live near a wastewater treatment plant? Specify the type and time of exposure..

    ....

12. Is there a person in your area (family members, neighbors, colleagues at work) with detected 1,2-dichloropropane in their blood or urine? ....

    ....

References

1. U.S. Department of Health and Human Services. Agency for Toxic Substances and Disease Registry. Toxicological profile for 1,2-dichloropropane. 2021, November.
2. IARC. Some halogenated hydrocarbons and pesticide exposures. IARC Monogr Eval Carcinog Risks Hum. 1986;41:1–407.
3. Chaoqun T. Application of 1,2-dichloropropane in coatings and ink industries. Paint Coatings Industry. 2008;38(8):48–50.
4. MHLW. Biliary tract cancer cases at printing plants in Japan. Japan: Ministry of Health, Labour and Welfare; 2013. Available from http://www.jisha.or.jp/english/pdf/Biliary_tract_cancer_cases_at_printing_plants_in_Japan.pdf. Accessed 3 Aug 2016.
5. OECD SIDS. 1,2-dichloropropane. CAS No. 78-87-5. SIDS initial assessment report from Siam 17. Arona, Italy, 11–15 November 2003. Organisation for Economic Co-operation and Development, Screening Information Dataset. United Nations Environment Programme Publications; 2003.
6. ACGIH. Propylene dichloride. Guide to occupational exposure values. Cincinnati: American Conference of Governmental Industrial Hygienists; 2006.
7. ECHA. 1,2-Dichloropropane. Substance information. Helsinki: European Chemicals Agency; 2016. Available from https://echa.europa.eu/substance-information/-/substanceinfo/100.001.048. Accessed 6 Jan 2015.

8. METI. Volumes of production and import of priority assessment chemical substances reported based on the act on the evaluation of chemical substances and regulation of their manufacture, etc. FY2011, announced on 25 March 2013. Tokyo: Ministry of Economy, Trade and Industry; 2013.

9. IARC. Some chemicals used as solvents and in polymer manufacture. IARC Monogr Eval Carcinog Risks Hum. 2017;110:1–289.

10. Radosavljević V. Urinarni markeri ekspozicije hemijskim kancerogenima—nove smernice u preventivnoj onkologiji (Urinary markers of exposure to chemical carcinogens—new guidelines in preventive oncology). Beograd: Medija centar „Odbrana"; 2024.

11. Radosavljevic V. Urinary markers/metabolites of exposure to chemical carcinogens—new possibilities in preventive oncology. Ecotoxicol Environ Saf. 2024; https://doi.org/10.1016/j.ecoenv.2023.115774.

17.1 Overview

Ethylene oxide is a raw material used as a base substance for the production of important derivatives, including di-, tri-, and poly(ethylene) glycols, cellulose and poly(propylene) glycol, ethylene glycol ethers, ethanol-amines, fatty alcohol products and fatty amines, and alkyl phenols [1–4]. A very small part of the production of ethylene oxide is used directly in gaseous form as a sterilization agent, fumigant, and insecticide (alone or in a mixture with nitrogen, carbon dioxide, or dichlorofluoromethane) [2, 5, 6]. Ethylene oxide is used to sterilize drugs, hospital equipment, disposable and reusable medical items, packaging materials, food, books, museum objects, scientific equipment, clothing, furs, wagons, airplanes, and beehives [7, 8].

Mainstream tobacco smoke contains 7 ng of ethylene oxide per cigarette [9]. Additional nonoccupational sources of ethylene oxide exposure are residues in spices, some food products [10], and skin care products, in very small amounts [11]. Ethylene oxide is produced during the burning of fossil fuel [7, 12].

There is a causal relationship between exposure to ethylene oxide and the occurrence of lymphatic and hematopoietic cancers (non-Hodgkin's lymphoma, multiple myeloma, and chronic lymphocytic leukemia) and breast cancer [13]. Its urinary carcinogen indicators are S-(2-hydroxyethyl)glutathione and N-acetyl-S-(2-hydroxyethyl)-L-cysteine (hydroxyethyl mercapturic acid [HEMA])—conjugates with glutathione, as well as ethylene glycol [14].

V. Radosavljevic, *Assessing Human Exposure to Key Chemical Carcinogens*, https://doi.org/10.1007/978-3-031-84441-6_17

Appendix: Exposure Evaluation Questionnaire

1. Did you work or live near chemical plants that produced of glycol ethers, polyglycol ethers, ethanolamines, ethoxylates, acrylonitrile, detergents, solvents, emulsifiers, fumigants, disinfection of food products? Specify the method, period (length of duration), and time (how long before sampling) of exposure...
....
....
....
....
....

2. Have you been exposed **tobacco smoke** and/or car exhaust fumes? Specify the method, period (length of duration), and time (how long before sampling) of exposure...
....
....
....
....

3. Have you participated in gas disinfection of medical material and/or medical equipment? Specify the method, period (length of duration), and time (how long before sampling) of exposure...
....
....
....

4. Do your close relatives (parents, brothers, sisters, children) have an increased level of ethylene oxide in their urine? ....
....

5. Have you been exposed to the smells of ripening fruits, vegetables, or grains? Specify the method, period (length of duration), and time (how long before sampling) of exposure...
....
....
....

6. Have you been exposed to the burning of fossil fuels (coal, oil, and their derivatives), pentane, or wood? Specify the method, period (length of duration), and time (how long before sampling) of exposure...
....
....
....

7. Have you been exposed to fires or frying in soybean oil? Specify the method, period (length of duration), and time (how long before sampling) of exposure...

8. Have you been exposed to antifreeze, glues, or working with plastic? Specify the method, period (length of duration), and time (how long before sampling) of exposure...

References

1. Lynch HN, Kozal JS, Russell AJ, Thompson WJ, Divis HR, Freid RD, Calabrese EJ, Mundt KA. Systematic review of the scientific evidence on ethylene oxide as a human carcinogen. Chem Biol Interact. 2022;364:110031.
2. Jones RR, Fisher JA, Medgyesi DN, Buller ID, Liao LM, Gierach G, Ward MH, Silverman DT. Ethylene oxide emissions and incident breast cancer and non-Hodgkin lymphoma in a US cohort. JNCI J Natl Cancer Inst. 2023;115(4):405–12. https://doi.org/10.1093/jnci/djad004.
3. Occupational Safety and Health Administration. Regulatory review of the occupational safety and health administration's ethylene oxide standard, 29 CFR 1910.1047. Washington, DC: Occupational Safety and Health Administration; 2005.
4. Devanney MT. CEH marketing research report—ethylene oxide (Abstract). Zurich: SRI Consulting; 2010.
5. Dever JP, George KF, Hoffman WC, Soo H. Ethylene oxide. In: Kirk-Othmer encyclopedia of chemical technology, vol. 10. New York: Wiley; 2004. p. 632–73. (Online).
6. Madrigal JM, Flory A, Fisher JA, Sharp E, Graubard BI, Ward MH, Jones RR. Sociodemographic inequities in the burden of carcinogenic industrial air emissions in the United States. JNCI J Natl Cancer Inst. 2024;00(0):1–8. https://doi.org/10.1093/jnci/djae001.
7. Kirman CR, Li AA, Sheehan PJ, Bus JS, Lewis RC, Hays SM. Ethylene oxide review: characterization of total exposure via endogenous and exogenous pathways and their implications to risk assessment and risk management. J Toxic Environ Health, Part B. 2021;24(1):1–29. https://doi.org/10.1080/10937404.2020.1852988.
8. Lacson J. CEH marketing research report—ethylene oxide. Zurich: SRI Consulting; 2003.
9. IARC. Tobacco smoke and involuntary smoking. IARC Monogr Eval Carcinog Risks Hum. 2004;83:1–1438.
10. Fowles J, Mitchell J, McGrath H. Assessment of cancer risk from ethylene oxide residues in spices imported into New Zealand. Food Chem Toxicol. 2001;39:1055–62.
11. Kreuzer PE. Permeation kinetics of ethylene oxide in gaseous form and dissolved other matrices through the skin of rats, hamsters and humans, GSF-Bericht 19/92. Neuherberg: GSF-Forschungszentrum fur Umwelt und Gesundheit; 1992.
12. WHO. Ethylene oxide, Concise international chemical assessment document 54. Geneva: WHO; 2003. Available at http://www.inchem.org

13. Radosavljević V. Urinarni markeri ekspozicije hemijskim kancerogenima—nove smernice u preventivnoj onkologiji (Urinary markers of exposure to chemical carcinogens—new guidelines in preventive oncology). Beograd: Medija centar „Odbrana"; 2024.
14. Radosavljevic V. Urinary markers/metabolites of exposure to chemical carcinogens—new possibilities in preventive oncology. Ecotoxicol Environ Saf. 2024; https://doi.org/10.1016/j.ecoenv.2023.115774.

18.1 Overview

Lindane is the γ-isomer of hexachlorocyclohexane (HHCH). There are several isomers of HHCH; β-, γ-, δ-, and ε-isomers are relatively stable. The γ-HHCH isomer has a very short half-life. There are pure and technical forms of lindane, with nearly pure lindane being γ-HHCH, while technical grade HHCH consists of 10–40% γ-HHCH and various other isomers. Only γ-HHCH has insecticidal properties [1] and is used worldwide as an insecticide [2]. Lindane is mobile, and as a result of atmospheric transport over long distances, it is deposited worldwide [3]. It has been measured in food, air, surface water, groundwater, sediments, soil, fish, wildlife, and humans [4, 5]. Current exposure of the general population occurs mainly through diet [6–8]. In most regions of the world, the proportion of human biological samples containing lindane at detectable levels is decreasing [4].

18.2 Occurrence in the Environment

Lindane does not occur naturally in the environment. Biodegradation is the dominant degradation process for γ-HHCH in aquatic systems and soil [9, 10].

18.2.1 Air

Air contamination with lindane is the result of pesticide application and dust emissions from production facilities [9, 11] Passive air sampling in 22 European countries in 2002 showed γ-HHCH concentrations from 1.1 to 65 pg/m^3, with the highest concentrations recorded in southern and eastern Europe, especially in Spain, parts of France, Italy, and the Balkan region [12]. According to the Global Passive Atmospheric Sampling Study (GAPS) between 2005 and 2008, different spatial and

V. Radosavljevic, *Assessing Human Exposure to Key Chemical Carcinogens*,
https://doi.org/10.1007/978-3-031-84441-6_18

temporal patterns show that pesticides such as γ-HHCH tend to be more prevalent in developing countries, especially in Asia. Samples taken from New Delhi, India, had the highest levels of γ-HHCH. In Europe, γ-HHCH levels are not evenly distributed, with samples from Paris having the highest levels. Levels of γ-HHCH are not very high in North and South America, which may reflect reduced use [13].

18.2.2 Water

Lindane enters water through agricultural and forestry use, precipitation, and to a lesser extent occasional pollution of wastewater from manufacturing plants [14, 15]. In India, a ban on the production of technical HHCH was enacted in 1997 [16, 17]. In Pakistan, between January and March 2013, the mean concentration of total HHCH was 3.31 ng/l for water collected from the Chenab River [18]. In southern China, mean HHCH levels in surface water decreased from 285 to 1.43 ng/l between 1999 and 2009 [19].

18.2.3 Soil and Dust

Lindane can be released into the soil by direct pesticide application [20, 21]. In Hong Kong, China, mean HHCH levels ranged from 1.14 to 26.8 µg/kg in samples from 12 different soil types [22]. Elsewhere in China, mean soil HHCH levels reported between 1999 and 2005 ranged from 3.65 to 5.92 ng/g dry weight [19]. The presence of γ-HHCH in house dust may contribute to human exposure. In a US household study where γ-HHCH in dust was measured at 5.85 ppb, the owner and his wife had elevated serum γ-HCH concentrations [9]. In Singapore, indoor dust samples from 31 homes contained γ-HHCH and β-HHCH at mean levels of 2.9 ng/g and 2.23 ng/g, respectively [23].

The largest number of data refer to non-Hodgkin's lymphoma (NHL) [24]. Its urinary metabolites are chlorophenols [25].

Appendix: Exposure Evaluation Questionnaire

1. Did you work in a pesticide factory or live near a pesticide factory? If so, which pesticides, for how long, and in which jobs?...
....
....

2. Have you used pesticides in plant protection or in agriculture? If so, which pesticides did you use, for how long, and for what purposes? ....
....
....

3. Have you worked in a pesticide dump or lived near a pesticide dump? If so, which pesticides, for how long, and in which jobs?....................
....

....

....

4. Did you work in a pesticide warehouse or live near a pesticide warehouse? Yes? If so, which pesticides, for how long, and in which jobs?....................

....

....

....

5. Have you worked on disinfection jobs? If so, which pesticides did you use, for how long, and in what specific jobs did you work?....................
....

....

....

6. Have you worked in pesticide destruction jobs or lived near places where pesticide destruction was carried out? If so, which pesticides, for how long, and in which jobs?....................

....

....

....

7. Did you consume grains (especially rice and corn) in large quantities during the week before giving your urine for analysis? If so, which cereals, for how long, and from which areas? ....

....

....

8. Did you consume a lot of fruit during the week before giving your urine for analysis? If so, which fruit, for how long, and from which areas?....................
....

....

....

9. Did you consume a lot of vegetables during the week before giving your urine for analysis? If yes, which fruit, for how long, and from which areas?..............
....

....

....

10. Did you consume milk and/or milk products in large quantities during the week before providing your urine for analysis? If so, which products, for how long, and from which areas?....................

....

....

....

11. Did you consume fish or seafood in large quantities during the week before providing your urine for analysis? If so, what kind of fish do they produce, for how long, and from which areas (rivers, seas, etc.)?...................................
....
....
....

12. Did you work in the wood industry or live near a wood industry factory? If so, which pesticides did you use, for how long, and in what jobs did you work?..
....
....
....

13. Have you worked in, or lived near, the recycling or wastewater treatment industry? If so, were pesticides or wood recycled (were pesticides also treated and which ones)? How long and in what jobs did you work?...................................
....
....
....

14. Did you grow and/or sell ornamental plants? If so, which pesticides did you use, for how long, and in what jobs did you work?...
....
....

15. Have you worked on the destruction of animal ectoparasites or lived near a livestock farm where the destruction of livestock ectoparasites was carried out? If so, which pesticides did you use, for how long, and in what jobs did you work?...
....
....

16. Have you used insecticides in the treatment of lice and scabies in humans? If so, which insecticides did you use, for how long, and in what jobs did you work?
....
....

17. Did you grow fodder plants or cultivate pastures? If so, what pesticides did you use, for how long, and what kind of work did you do?
....
....

18. Did you work in the plastics industry or live near such places, and were insecticides used there and which ones? If so, which pesticides, how long, and in what jobs did you work?...
....
....
....

19. Have you used insecticides for military purposes? If so, which insecticides, how long were they used, and what jobs did you work in?.................................. ....

20. Have you been exposed to high temperatures for several hours on surfaces where pesticides were once intensively used (two or three decades ago)? If so, how long were you exposed to and to how high temperatures? What pesticides were used and for how long on such land? ....

21. Did you consume a lot of water during the week before giving your urine for analysis? If so, is that water from arterial wells on agricultural land? How long and in what quantity did you consume it? ....

22. Did you consume animal fat in a larger amount during the week before giving your urine for analysis? If so, how long and in what quantity did you consume them? ....

23. Were there floods in your area? If so, when and where did the tidal wave come from? ....

24. Are there any lymphoma patients in your area?.. ....

25. Do you live in an urban, semi-urban, or rural settlement? ....

26. Do you use insecticides in your household? Which, when, in which places, and under what conditions? ....

27. Is there an intensive use of insecticides/pesticides in the area where you lived or live? If there is, when is it applied, for how long, and for what purposes? ....

28. Do you often consume wine and/or fruit juices? If you consume them, how often and in what quantity? ....

References

1. Brooks GC. Chlorinated insecticides: retrospect and prospect. In: Plimmer JR, editor. Pesticide chemistry in the 20th century, ACS symposium series. Washington, DC: American Chemical Society; 1977. p. 1–19.
2. Vijgen J, de Borst B, Weber R, Stobiecki T, Forter M. HCH and lindane contaminated sites: European and global need for a permanent solution for a long-time neglected issue. Environ Pollut. 2019;248:696e705. https://doi.org/10.1016/j.envpol.2019.02.029.
3. Alehashem M, Peters R, Fajana HO, Eslamizad S, Hogan N, Hecker M, Siciliano SD. Herbicides and pesticides synergistically interact at low concentrations in complex mixtures. Chemosphere. 2024; https://doi.org/10.1016/j.chemosphere.2024.141431.
4. Vijgen J, Fokke B, van de Coterlet G, Amstaetter K, Sancho J, Bensaïah C, Weber R. European cooperation to tackle the legacies of hexachlorocyclohexane (HCH) and lindane. Emerg Contam. 2022;8:97e112.
5. Ting X, Miao J, Chen Y, Yin D, Shuangqing H, Daniel Sheng G. The long-term environmental risks from the aging of organochlorine pesticide lindane. Environ Int. 2020;141:105778.
6. David BC, Tutuwa JA, Tadawu RH, Jesse PS, Ogu EO, Sunday OG, Nuhu I, Haruna PG. Investigation of organochlorines residue in stored cereals from some selected markets in Jalingo, Nigeria. Int J Educ Cult Soc. 2024;2(1):1–14. https://doi.org/10.58578/IJECS.v2i1.2406.
7. Faraj TK, EL-Saeid MH, Najim MMM, Chieb M. The impact of pesticide residues on soil health for sustainable vegetable production in arid areas. Separations. 2024;11:46. https://doi.org/10.3390/separations11020046.
8. Miclean M, Levei EA, Cadar O. Organochlorine pesticides in dairy cows' diet and the carryover into Milk in NW Romania. Sustain For. 2024;16:434. https://doi.org/10.3390/su16010434.
9. ATSDR. Toxicological profile for alpha-, beta-, gamma-, and delta-hexachlorocyclohexane. Atlanta: Agency for Toxic Substances and Disease Registry; 2005. Available from http://www.atsdr.cdc.gov/toxprofiles/tp43.pdf
10. Navarro I, de la Torre A, Sanz P, Arjol MA, Fernández J, Martínez MA. Organochlorine pesticides air monitoring near a historical lindane production site in Spain. Sci Total Environ. 2019;670:1001–7. https://doi.org/10.1016/j.scitotenv.2019.03.313.
11. Tadevosyan NS, Kirakosyan GV, Muradyan SA, Poghosyan SB, Khachatryan BG. Relationship between respiratory morbidity and environmental exposure to organochlorine pesticides in Armenia. J Health Pollut. 2021;11(31):210904.
12. Jaward FM, Farrar NJ, Harner T, Sweetman AJ, Jones KC. Passive air sampling of PCBs, PBDEs, and organochlorine pesticides across Europe. Environ Sci Technol. 2004;38(1):34–41.
13. Shunthirasingham C, Oyiliagu CE, Cao X, Gouin T, Wania F, Lee SC, et al. Spatial and temporal pattern of pesticides in the global atmosphere. J Environ Monit. 2010;12(9):1650–7.
14. WHO. Lindane in drinking-water. Background document for development of WHO Guidelines for Drinking-water Quality, WHO/SDE/WSH/03.04/102. Geneva: World Health Organization; 2004. Available from http://www.who.int/water_sanitation_health/dwq/chemicals/lindane.pdf
15. Pan H, Lei H, He X, Xi B, Qigong X. Spatial distribution of organochlorine and organophosphorus pesticides in soil-groundwater systems and their associated risks in the middle reaches of the Yangtze River Basin. Environ Geochem Health. 2019;41:1833–45. https://doi.org/10.1007/s10653-017-9970-1.
16. Sharma BM, Bharat GK, Tayal S, Nizzetto L, Cupr P, Larssen T. Environment and human exposure to persistent organic pollutants (POPs) in India: a systematic review of recent and historical data. Environ Int. 2014;66:48–64.
17. Adithya S, Jayaraman RS, Krishnan A, Malolan R, Gopinath KP, Arun J, Kim W, Govarthanan M. A critical review on the formation, fate and degradation of the persistent organic pollutant hexachlorocyclohexane in water systems and waste streams. Chemosphere. 2021;271:129866. https://doi.org/10.1016/j.chemosphere.2021.129866.

18. Mahmood A, Malik RN, Li J, Zhang G. Levels, distribution pattern and ecological risk assessment of organochlorines pesticides (OCPs) in water and sediments from two tributaries of the Chenab River, Pakistan. Ecotoxicology. 2014;23(9):1713–21.

19. Zhang K, Wei YL, Zeng EY. A review of environmental and human exposure to persistent organic pollutants in the Pearl River Delta, South China. Sci Total Environ. 2013;463-464:1093–110.

20. Iribarne-Duran LM, Castillero-Rosales I, Peinado FM, Artacho-Cordon F, Molina-Molina JM, Medianero E, Nicolas-Delgado SI, Sanchez-Pinzon L, Núnez-Samudio V, Vela-Soria F, Olea N, Alvarado-Gonzalez NE. Placental concentrations of xenoestrogenic organochlorine pesticides and polychlorinated biphenyls and assessment of their xenoestrogenicity in the PA-MAMI mother-child cohort. Environ Res. 2024;241:117622.

21. Anand N, Chakraborty P, Ray S. Human exposure to organochlorine, pyrethroid and neonicotinoid pesticides: comparison between urban and semi-urban regions of India. Environ Pollut. 2021;270:116156. https://doi.org/10.1016/j.envpol.2020.116156.

22. Man YB, Chow KL, Wang HS, Lau KY, Sun XL, Wu SC, et al. Health risk assessment of organochlorine pesticides with emphasis on DDTs and HCHs in abandoned agricultural soils. J Environ Monit. 2011;13(8):2250–9.

23. Tan J, Cheng SM, Loganath A, Chong YS, Obbard JP. Selected organochlorine pesticide and polychlorinated biphenyl residues in house dust in Singapore. Chemosphere. 2007;68(9):1675–82.

24. Radosavljević V. Urinarni markeri ekspozicije hemijskim kancerogenima—nove smernice u preventivnoj onkologiji (Urinary markers of exposure to chemical carcinogens—new guidelines in preventive oncology). Beograd: Medija centar „Odbrana“; 2024.

25. Radosavljevic V. Urinary markers/metabolites of exposure to chemical carcinogens—new possibilities in preventive oncology. Ecotoxicol Environ Saf. 2024; https://doi.org/10.1016/j.ecoenv.2023.115774.

Human Exposure to 4,4′-Methylenebis (2-Chloroaniline)

19.1 Overview

4,4′-Methylenebis(2-chloroaniline) (eng. 4,4′-methylenebis(2-chloroaniline), abbreviated MOCA) is used for coatings and cast polyurethanes [1, 2]. The general population can be exposed to MOCA if they live or spend time on land contaminated with it. Drinking water or eating certain types of plants (root crops) grown in an area contaminated with MOCA can significantly expose the population. Even immediate family members of MOCA-exposed workers may be affected by MOCA concentrations in urine of up to 15 µg/l.

There is no commercial use of pure 4,4′-methylenebis(2-chloroaniline) except for academic laboratory work [3], but 4,4′-methylenebis(2-chloroaniline) accounts for up to 92% of the commercial production of MOCA. MOCA production in the USA ceased in 1982 [4] and in the United Kingdom in 1987, but increased quantities were imported from Taiwan [5] and some other countries [6]. Available information indicated that 4,4′-methylenebis(2-chloroaniline) was produced and/or shipped to the Hong Kong Special Administrative Region of the People's Republic of China, Taiwan, Japan, South Africa, Germany, Switzerland, and the USA [7]. MOCA is not known as a natural product. It is rapidly absorbed into the soil and exists mostly in a covalently bound state [8]. It is used as a curing agent for isocyanate-containing polymers, and only about 1% is used in epoxy/epoxy-urethane resin blends, for curing castable liquid polyurethane elastomers. MBOCA-cured polyurethanes have been used to produce shoe soles, rolls for postage stamp machines, cutting bars in plywood manufacturing, rolls and belt drives in cameras, computers, wheels and pulleys for escalators and elevators, in the manufacture of gun mounts, jet engine turbine blades, radar systems, components in home appliances, as a wiring patting, ball seals on nuclear submarines, positioning strips in "Poseidon" missiles, and castable urethane rubber products, such as absorption pads, conveyor belts, and encapsulation of electric components [9–12].

V. Radosavljevic, *Assessing Human Exposure to Key Chemical Carcinogens*, https://doi.org/10.1007/978-3-031-84441-6_19

MOCA causes an increased incidence of bladder cancers in exposed workers [13]. MOCA and conjugates are urinary carcinogen biomarkers for 4,4′-methylenebis(2-chloroaniline) [14].

Appendix: Exposure Evaluation Questionnaire

1. Did you work in the polyurethane industry or live near such places, or places where polyurethane products were disposed/stored? If so, how long did you work/live in such places and what jobs did you work in the polyurethane industry? ....
....
....
....

2. Did you work in the industry of urethane rubber, industrial rubber, conveyor belts, or absorbent materials (pads) or lived near such places, or places where raw materials or finished products of the mentioned industries were stored? If so, how long have you worked/lived in such places and what jobs have you held in the mentioned industries? ....
....
....
....
....

3. Have you worked in the waste water industry or lived near such places? If so, how long have you worked/lived in such places and what jobs have you held in the waste water industry? ....
....
....

4. Have you worked in the industry of sealants (for wood or roof structures), urethane resins, urethane resins, chipboard, insulating materials for the electrical industry, ball seals, turbines and jet engines, weapon mounts, or positioning tapes? If so, how long have you worked/lived in such places and what jobs have you held in the mentioned industries? ....
....
....
....
....

5. Have you worked in landfills or lived near such places? If so, how long did you work/live in such places and what jobs did you do?...
....
....
....
....
....

6. During the last week before giving the sample for analysis, did you consume turnips, cabbage, beans, turnips, cane sugar, or cucumber? If so, how often and in what quantity? ....
....
....
....

7. Have you worked in the ski equipment industry (rubber ski boots) or lived near such places? If so, how long have you worked/lived in such places and what jobs did you do?..
....

8. Did you work in shipyards? If so, how long have you worked in such places (watering and shaping masses/spaces) and what jobs did you do?
....
....
....
....

9. Have you worked in laboratories where 4,4′-methylenebis(2-chloroaniline) was used? If so, how long have you worked in such places and what jobs did you do?...
....
....

10. Did you work in the production of gears, polyurethane moldings or lived near such places? If so, how long have you worked/lived in such places and what jobs did you do? ....
....

11. Have you worked in the production of shoe soles, rollers and belt drives in cameras, or wheels and pulleys for escalators and elevators? If so, how long have you worked/lived in such places and what jobs did you do?...............................
....
....

References

1. Agency for Toxic Substances and Disease Registry. 4,4′-methylenebis(2-chloroaniline) (MBOCA). Page last reviewed: February 10, 2021. https://wwwn.cdc.gov/TSP/substances/ToxSubstance.aspx?toxid=209. Accessed 3 July 2024.
2. Australian Government. Department of Climate Change, Energy, the Environment and Water. 4,4′-methylene-bis(2-chloroaniline) (MOCA). Last updated: 30 June 2022. https://www.dcceew.gov.au/environment/protection/npi/substances/fact-sheets/44-methylene-bis2-chloroaniline-moca
3. ATSDR. Toxicological profile For 4,4′-methylenebis(2-chloroaniline) MBOCA; 1994. p. 120.

4. NTP. 4,4′-methylenebis(2-chloroaniline) CAS No. 101-14-4. Report on Carcinogens. 11th ed. U.S. Department of Health and Human Services, Public Health Service, National Toxicology Program, 2005. http://ntp.niehs.nih.gov/ntp/roc/eleventh/profiles/s073dmob.pdf

5. Chen HI, Liou SH, Loh CH, et al. Bladder cancer screening and monitoring of 4,4′-methylenebis(2-chloroaniline) exposure among workers in Taiwan. Urology. 2005;66:305–10.

6. Cocker J, Cain JR, Baldwin P, et al. A survey of occupational exposure to 4,4′-methylenebis (2-chloroaniline) (MbOCA) in the UK. Ann Occup Hyg. 2009;53:499–507.

7. Chemical Sources International. ChemSources database. 2008. http://db2.chemsources.com

8. Voorman R, Penner D. Fate of MBOCA (4,4′-methylene-bis(2-chloroaniline)) in soil. Arch Environ Contam Toxicol. 1986;15:595–602.

9. U.S. Department of Health and Human Services. Agency for Toxic Substances and Disease Registry. Toxicological profile for 4,4′-methylenebis(2-chloroaniline) (MBOCA), 2017, October.

10. European Chemicals Agency (ECHA). Committee for Risk Assessment (RAC) Opinion on 4,4′-methylene-bis-[2-chloroaniline] (MOCA). EC number: 202–918-9. CAS number: 101-14-4. Adopted 29 May 2017.

11. HBM4EU. Substance report. Anilines and Diisocyanates. 2022, June.

12. Shankar K, Fung V, Seneviratne M, O'Donnell GE. Exposure to 4,4′-methylene *bis*(2-chloroaniline) (MbOCA) in New South Wales, Australia. J Occup Health. 2017;59:296–303.

13. Radosavljević V. Urinarni markeri ekspozicije hemijskim kancerogenima—nove smernice u preventivnoj onkologiji (Urinary markers of exposure to chemical carcinogens—new guidelines in preventive oncology). Beograd: Medija centar „Odbrana"; 2024.

14. Radosavljevic V. Urinary markers/metabolites of exposure to chemical carcinogens—new possibilities in preventive oncology. Ecotoxicol Environ Saf. 2024; https://doi.org/10.1016/j.ecoenv.2023.115774.

20.1 Overview

2-Naphthylamine is used only in laboratory research. It is formed during the pyrolysis of organic substances containing nitrogen and as such can occur in nature [1]. 2-NA has been detected in hair dyes as well as rubber antioxidants at levels of 0.25% [2]. Several dye and pigment intermediates, paperboards, have been shown to contain small amounts of 2-naphthylamine [3, 4].

The main sources of exposure of the general population are from the environment, 2-naphthylamine and 2-nitronaphthalene, tobacco smoke, fumes from cooking oil, lubricants for automobile engines, in brake fluids, oils, contact with some types of dyes, and hair dyes contaminated with 2-NA [5–8]. 2-Naphthylamine and 4-aminobiphenyls are degraded in urine within a few hours, which explains why they are difficult to detect in such samples [3].

2-Naphthylamine causes bladder cancer in humans, especially in Caucasians [5]. Its urinary metabolites are 2-naphthylamine, N-(2-naphthyl)-hydroxylamine, bis-(2-amino1-naphthyl) phosphate, 2-aminobiphenyl, and 4-aminobiphenyl [9].

Appendix: Exposure Evaluation Questionnaire

1. Are you a smoker or are you exposed to tobacco smoke? If so, when and how much did you smoke or were you exposed to tobacco smoke? ....
....
....
....

V. Radosavljevic, *Assessing Human Exposure to Key Chemical Carcinogens*, https://doi.org/10.1007/978-3-031-84441-6_20

2. Do you wear skin-tight clothing dyed with synthetic dyes? If you wear it, state when you wear it and for how long?..
....
....
....

3. If you wear clothes that stick to your skin, dyed with synthetic dyes, do you know from which country such clothes come from or who is the manufacturer? ....
....
....

4. Do you work or live near paint, rubber, motor lubricants and oil, or brake oil factories? If so, how long did you work/live in such places and what jobs did you do? ....
....
....
....
....

5. Do you use electronic cigarettes or are you exposed to their smoke? If so, when and how much did you smoke electronic cigarettes or were you exposed to their smoke? ....
....
....

6. Do you work or live near cardboard or cardboard packaging factories? If so, how long did you work/live in such places and what jobs did you do?
....
....
....
....

7. Do you often use food from cardboard packaging? If so, state when you consumed it and for how long? ....
....
....
....

References

1. Talukder M, Kates CR. Naphthalene derivatives. In: Kirk Othmer encyclopedia of chemical technology. Hoboken: Wiley; 2000.
2. Veys CA. Bladder tumours in rubber workers: a factory study 1946-1995. Occup Med (Lond). 2004;54:322–9.
3. IARC. Some aromatic amines, organic dyes, and related exposures. IARC Monogr Eval Carcinog Risks Hum. 2010;99:1–706.
4. Parigoridi I-E, Tsoumani E, Akrida-Demertzi K, Demertzis PG. Determination of nitrogen-containing organic compounds in commercially available recycled cardboards intended for food contact applications. Sustain Chem Pharm. 2024;38:101468. https://doi.org/10.1016/j.scp.2024.101468.

5. Radosavljević V. Urinarni markeri ekspozicije hemijskim kancerogenima—nove smernice u preventivnoj onkologiji (Urinary markers of exposure to chemical carcinogens—new guidelines in preventive oncology). Beograd: Medija centar „Odbrana"; 2024.
6. Jeżewska A, Kondej D. Determination of phenyl(2-naphthyl)amine concentrations in the working environment air using HPLC-FLD technique. Med Pr Work Health Saf. 2022;73(1):25–31. https://doi.org/10.13075/mp.5893.01152.
7. Golka K, Bolt HM, Drexler H, Hartwig A, MAK Commission. 2-naphthylamine—addendum for re-evaluation of study results in biological material. Assessment values in biological material—translation of the German version from 2021. MAK Collect Occup Health Saf. 2021;6(2):Doc041. https://doi.org/10.34865/bb9159e6_2ad.
8. Souza MCO, Gonzalez N, Rovira J, Herrero M, Marques M, Nadal M, Barbosa F Jr, Domingo JL. Assessment of urinary aromatic amines in Brazilian pregnant women and association with DNA damage: influence of genetic diversity, lifestyle, and environmental and socioeconomic factors. Environ Pollut. 2023;335:122366. https://doi.org/10.1016/j.envpol.2023.122366.
9. Radosavljevic V. Urinary markers/metabolites of exposure to chemical carcinogens—new possibilities in preventive oncology. Ecotoxicol Environ Saf. 2024; https://doi.org/10.1016/j.ecoenv.2023.115774.

21.1 Overview

Orthotoluidine is used as an intermediate in the synthesis of herbicides, more than 90 colors and pigments, for synthetic rubber, pharmaceutical products, pesticides, and in the clinical laboratory as an ingredient in reagents for glucose analysis and tissue staining [1–5].

Significant nonoccupational exposure to orthotoluidine may result from the use of some hair dyes, the local anesthetic prilocaine, or tobacco smoke [1, 3, 6]. It was detected in surface waters and industrial effluents [5–8]. Its levels were very low in vegetables (kale, celery, carrots, black tea) [4], even in breast milk [9].

Orthotoluidine causes bladder cancer [10–13]. Its urinary metabolites are ortho-toluidine and its conjugates and N-acetyl-ortho-toluidine [14].

Appendix: Exposure Evaluation Questionnaire

1. Do you work or live near rubber or paint and varnish factories? If so, how long did you work/live in such places and what jobs did you do?

   ....

   ....

   ....

   ....

2. Do you work in the production of ortho-toluidine? If you work, how long have you worked and what jobs have you held? ....

   ....

   ....

   ....

V. Radosavljevic, *Assessing Human Exposure to Key Chemical Carcinogens,*
https://doi.org/10.1007/978-3-031-84441-6_21

3. Do you work or live near organic dye or pigment factories? If so, how long did
   you work/live in such places and what jobs did you do?
   ....
   ....
   ....
   ....

4. Do you work or live near artificial resin or herbicide factories? If so, how long
   did you work/live in such places and what jobs did you do?
   ....
   ....
   ....
   ....

5. Do you work or live near indigodye or photographic dye factories? If so, how
   long did you work/live in such places and what jobs did you do?
   ....
   ....
   ....
   ....

6. Are you a smoker or do you stay in rooms where there is tobacco smoke? If so,
   how long have you worked/lived in such places? ....
   ....
   ....
   ....
   ....

7. Do you stay in rooms where there was a lot of tobacco smoke before? If so, how
   long have you worked/lived in such places? ....
   ....
   ....

8. Do you work or live near a wastewater treatment plant? If so, how long did you
   work/live in such places and what jobs did you do?
   ....
   ....
   ....
   ....

9. Do you work or stay in premises where tissue staining for microscopic preparations is performed? If so, how long have you worked in such places? ....
   ....
   ....
   ....
   ....

10. Do you work or stay in premises where blood or urine glucose analyzes are
    performed? If so, how long have you worked in such places? ....
    ....
    ....

11. Do you work or stay in premises where dental anesthetics (prilocaine) are applied? If so, how long have you worked in such places? ....
....
....

12. Do you have tattoos and when did you get them? Have you tattooed other people? If so, how long have you worked in such places?
....
....
....
....

13. Do you work or stay in premises where hair dyes or varnishes are used? If so, how long did you work/stay in such places? ....
....
....
....
....

14. Do you work or stay in premises where hair dyes are used? If so, how long did you work/stay in such places? ....
....
....

References

1. Santonen T, Mahiout S, Alvito P, Apel P, Bessems J, Bil W, Borges T, Stephan Bose-O'Reilly, Buekers J, Portilla AIC, Calvo AC, de Alba Gonzalez M, Domínguez-Morueco N, L'opez ME, Falnoga I, Gerofke A, del Carmen Gonzalez Caballero M, Horvat M, Huuskonen P, Kadikis N, Kolossa-Gehring M, Lange R, Louro H, Martins C, Meslin M, Niemann L, Díaz SP, Plichta V, Porras SP, Rousselle C, Scholten B, Silva MJ, Slejkovec Z, Tratnik JS, Joksic AS, Tarazona JV, Uhl M, Van Nieuwenhuyse A, Viegas S, Vinggaard AM, Woutersen M, Schoeters G. How to use human biomonitoring in chemical risk assessment: methodological aspects, recommendations, and lessons learned from HBM4EU. Int J Hyg Environ Health. 2023;249:114139. https://doi.org/10.1016/j.ijheh.2023.114139.
2. Huuskonen P, Karakitsios S, Scholten B, Westerhout J, Sarigiannis DA, Santonen T. Health risk assessment of ortho-toluidine utilising human biomonitoring data of workers and the general population. Toxics. 2022;10:217. https://doi.org/10.3390/toxics10050217.
3. National Toxicology Program, Department of Health and Human Services. o-Toluidine. 15th report on carcinogens. 2021.
4. IARC. Chemical agents and related occupations. IARC Monogr Eval Carcinog Risks Hum. 2012;100F:1–628.
5. NTP. o-toluidine and o-toluidine hydrochloride. Rep Carcinog. 2004;11:258–9.
6. Soleimani F, Masjedi MR, Tangestani M, Arfaeinia H, Dobaradaran S, Farhadi A, Afrashteh S, Mallaki R, Vakilabadi DR. Primary aromatic amines (PAAs) in third-hand smoke collected from waterpipe/cigarette cafés: level and exposure assessment. Arab J Chem. 2024;17:105587. https://doi.org/10.1016/j.arabjc.2023.105587.
7. EPA. Chemical Hazard Information Profile (CHIP): ortho-toluidine; ortho-toluidine hydrochloride. Washington, DC: Office of Pesticide Programs and Toxic Substances; 1984.

8. Shokri A, Mahanpoor K. Removal of ortho-toluidine from industrial wastewater by UV/TiO2 process. J Chem Health Risks. 2016;6(3):213–23.
9. De Bruin LS, Pawliszyn JB, Josephy PD. Detection of monocyclic aromatic amines, possible mammary carcinogens, in human milk. Chem Res Toxicol. 1999;12:78–82.
10. Suzuki S, Gi M, Komiya M, Obikane A, Vachiraarunwong A, Fujioka M, Kakehashi A, Totsuka Y, Wanibuchi H. Evaluation of the mechanisms involved in the development of bladder toxicity following exposure to occupational bladder cancer causative chemicals using DNA adductome analysis. Biomol Ther. 2024;14:36. https://doi.org/10.3390/biom14010036.
11. Hosseini B, Zendehdel K, Bouaoun L, et al. Bladder cancer risk in relation to occupations held in a nationwide case-control study in Iran. Int J Cancer. 2023;153(4):765–74. https://doi.org/10.1002/ijc.34560.
12. Nakano M, Omae K, Takebayashi T, Tanaka S, Koda S. An epidemic of bladder cancer: ten cases of bladder cancer in male Japanese workers exposed to *ortho*-toluidine. J Occup Health. 2018;60(4):307–11. https://doi.org/10.1539/joh.2017-0220-OA.
13. Radosavljević V. Urinarni markeri ekspozicije hemijskim kancerogenima—nove smernice u preventivnoj onkologiji (Urinary markers of exposure to chemical carcinogens—new guidelines in preventive oncology). Beograd: Medija centar „Odbrana"; 2024.
14. Radosavljevic V. Urinary markers/metabolites of exposure to chemical carcinogens—new possibilities in preventive oncology. Ecotoxicol Environ Saf. 2024; https://doi.org/10.1016/j.ecoenv.2023.115774.

22.1 Overview

The production of pentachlorophenol leads to contamination with dioxins (2,3,7,8-tetrachlorodibenzo-para-dioxin [THDD]), furans, hexachlorobenzene (hexachlorodibenzo-para-dioxin), hexachlorodibenzo-para-dioxin (HHDD), para-dioxin (PD), and octachlorodibenzo-para-dioxin (OHDD). Accordingly, commercial pentachlorophenol is approximately 90% pentachlorophenol and 10% impurities [1, 2]. In Europe, pentachlorophenol production existed in Poland, Germany, the Netherlands, Switzerland, the United Kingdom, Spain, and France and ceased in most countries in 1992 [3], except in Spain, in 2003 [2]. China is probably the largest producer of pentachlorophenol in the world [2].

The largest application of pentachlorophenol is as a wood preservative [2], for which it has been discontinued in the European Union since 2009 [2]. However, pentachlorophenol has been widely used as an herbicide, germicide, fungicide, defoliant, wood preservative, algicide, and molluscicide [4]. Because of this, it became ubiquitous and could be found in brick walls, adhesives, insulation, leather, paints, canvas, textiles (not intended for clothing), railway sleepers, wooden piles, fence posts and lumber/wood for construction, ropes, etc. [1, 2, 5–7]. Continued use in Asia to clean ponds against schistosomiasis vectors has been reported. Despite the restrictions in 2016, almost 30 companies were registered for the production of pentachlorophenol: in the USA (10), the United Kingdom (3), Mexico (2), Germany (2), Switzerland (2), Canada (1), South Africa (1), India (1), Israel (1), Netherlands (1), China (2), and Japan (1) [8].

V. Radosavljevic, *Assessing Human Exposure to Key Chemical Carcinogens*,
https://doi.org/10.1007/978-3-031-84441-6_22

22.2   Exposure of the General Population

As a porous organic pollutant, pentachlorophenol persists long after its use [2, 9]. Thus, the general population could be exposed through wood treated with pentachlorophenol [10, 11] or other listed products (especially through contact with skin and textiles treated with pentachlorophenol; for example, leather car seats in hot weather) [12]; from food, soil, and contaminated water; and emissions from incinerators [2, 13, 14]. Pentachlorophenol is mainly absorbed in the soil (96.5%) and accumulates in the food chain (cereals, vegetables, fruits) [10, 11].

22.2.1 Water

Pentachlorophenol has low solubility in water [12, 15]. Concentrations in tap and well water in China and Poland ranged from 0.01 to 3.27 µg/l [7, 16], while river water samples had concentrations of pentachlorophenol up to 640 µg/l [16]. Seawater samples from Belgium, France, Germany, the Netherlands, and the United Kingdom contained pentachlorophenol at concentrations of 0.01–0.17 µg/l [17].

22.2.2 Sediment and Soil

Of the 37 sites tested in China, mean concentrations of pentachlorophenol in soil were <10 µg/kg dry weight for 29 sites, between 10 and 63 µg/kg for seven sites, and one site had a mean concentration of 15,850 µg/kg [7].

22.2.3 Air

In 30 air samples collected in Canada, concentrations of pentachlorophenol ranged from 0.23 ng/m^3 in Waskesiu to 1.53 ng/m^3 in Yellowknife [18]. Pentachlorophenol was detected in 96% of 861 dust samples from German homes (mean concentration 0.3 µg/g; range 0.03–30.9 µg/g) [19, 20]. Analyses of dust samples from homes and institutions day cares in North Carolina and Ohio, USA, from 2000 to 2001, showed the presence of pentachlorophenol in more than 50% of indoor air samples [15]. A study conducted in California, USA, from 2001 to 2006, showed the arithmetic mean concentration of pentachlorophenol of 199 ng/g in 94% of household dust samples taken from rooms where children spend most of their time [21].

22.2.4 Food

Very low concentrations of pentachlorophenol have been reported in aquatic organisms, up to 172 µg/kg raw weight [7, 22]. Pentachlorophenol was detected in samples of pork, beef, chicken, eggs [23], and chicken coop material (concentrations 11 ± 2.8 µg/kg) [24, 25]. It was found in about 20% of the solid food samples of 257 children in the USA [26]. Concentrations of pentachlorophenol in red wine ranged from 12 to 123 ng/l [27] and probably originate from oak barrels used for aging wine and other spirits (concentrations in oak barrels 5–120 µg/g) [26].

Pentachlorophenol causes non-Hodgkin's lymphoma in humans [28]. Its urinary metabolites are pentachlorophenol and nonspecific tetrachloro-p-hydroquinone (TCHQ) [29].

Appendix: Exposure Evaluation Questionnaire

1. During the last month, have you used (or been exposed to) bactericides, fungicides, herbicides, algicides, defoliants, or tree protection agents? If so, when was it and to what extent? ....
   ....
   ....
   ....
   ....

2. Do you work in the wood industry (carpentry) or in the industry of wood protection chemicals? Do you live near a wood industry or near a wood protection chemical industry? If so, when was it, how long was it, and to what extent were you exposed to the chemicals? ....
   ....
   ....
   ....
   ....
   ....

3. During the last week, have you consumed a large amount of pork, chicken, or river fish? If so, when was it, how many times did you consume it, and in what quantity? ....
   ....
   ....
   ....
   ....
   ....

4. During the last week, have you consumed a large amount of beef, mutton, offal, eggs, or poultry? If so, when was it, how many times did you consume it, and in what quantity? ....
   ....
   ....
   ....
   ....
   ....

5. Did you work in a fish farm? If so, when, in what jobs, and for how long?..........
....
....

6. Did you work in the furniture industry? If so, when, in what jobs, and for how long? ....
....
....
....

7. During the last week, have you consumed a large amount of seafood (shellfish, crabs, shrimps)? If so, when was it, how many times did you consume it, and in what quantity? ....
....
....
....
....
....

8. Have you worked in the industry: leather, paper, or shipyards? If so, when, in what jobs, and for how long?...
....
....
....

9. Have there been people in your environment (family members, neighbors, colleagues at work, etc.) suffering from non-Hodgkin's lymphoma? If so, who got sick and when? ....
....
....

10. Is your diet rich in animal fats? Have you consumed a large amount of animal fat during the last week? If so, when and how much?
....
....
....
....

11. Have you worked in rice fields or in swampy conditions? If so, when, in what jobs, and for how long?...
....
....
....

12. Did you work in metal mines? If so, in which mines, when, on which jobs, and for how long?...
....
....
....

13. During the last week, did you consume a large amount of river fish or fish from a pond? If so, when was it, how many times did you consume it, and in what quantity? ....

....

....

14. Have you worked or lived near a wastewater treatment plant? If so, in which plants, when, in which jobs, and for how long?.................................

....

....

15. During the last week, have you consumed a large quantity of onions, lettuce, or other bulbous vegetables? If so, when was it, how many times did you consume it, and in what quantity? ....

....

....

16. During the last week, did you consume a large amount of milk and milk products? If so, when was it, how many times did you consume it, and in what quantity? ....

....

....

References

1. EPA. Toxicological review of pentachlorophenol (CAS No. 87-86-5). In support of summary information on the Integrated Risk Information System (IRIS). Washington, DC: United States Environmental Protection Agency; 2010.
2. United Nations. Exploration of management options por pentachlorophenol (PCP). Paper for the 8th meeting of the UNECE CLRTAP Task Force on Persistent Organic Pollutants. Montreal, 18–20 May 2010; 2010.
3. OSPAR. Pentachlorophenol, Hazardous substances series. OSPAR Commission 2001 (2004 Update). London: Committee on the Convention for the Protection of the Marine Environment of the North-East Atlantic; 2004. Available from http://www.ospar.org/documents?v=6921
4. Sun Y, Liu Z, Xia W, He Z, Wan Y. Urinary pentachlorophenol in general population of central China: reproducibility, predictors, and associations with oxidative stress biomarkers. Environ Sci Pollut Res. 2023;30:37598–606. https://doi.org/10.1007/s11356-022-24802-y.
5. NTP. NTP toxicology and carcinogenesis studies of pentachlorophenol (CAS No. 87-86-5) in F344/N rats (feed studies). Natl Toxicol Program Tech Rep Ser. 1999;483:1–182.
6. CAREX Canada. Pentachlorophenol. Profile. Vancouver: CAREX Canada; 2009. Available from http://www.carexcanada.ca/en/pentachlorophenol/
7. Zheng W, Yu H, Wang X, Qu W. Systematic review of pentachlorophenol occurrence in the environment and in humans in China: not a negligible health risk due to the re-emergence of schistosomiasis. Environ Int. 2012;42:105–16.
8. Sources C. Pentachlorophenol. Chem sources online. Pendleton: Chemical Sources International, Inc; 2016. Available from http://www.chemsources.com. Accessed Oct 2016.

9. Favaro G, De Leo D, Pastore P, Magno F, Ballardin A. Quantitative determination of chlorophenols in leather by pressurized liquid extraction and liquid chromatography with diode-array detection. J Chromatogr A. 2008;1177(1):36–42.

10. Hattemer-Frey HA, Travis CC. Pentachlorophenol: environmental partitioning and human exposure. Arch Environ Contam Toxicol. 1989;18(4):482–9.

11. Coad S, Newhook RC. PCP exposure for the Canadian general population: a multimedia analysis. J Expo Anal Environ Epidemiol. 1992;2(4):391–413.

12. Choudhary AK, Kumar S, Sharma C. Removal of chlorophenolics from pulp and paper mill wastewater through constructed wetland. Water Environ Res. 2013;85(1):54–62.

13. Yang F, Wan Y, Wang Y, Li S, Xu S, Xia W. Occurrence of pentachlorophenol in surface water from the upper to lower reaches of the Yangtze River and treated water in Wuhan, China. Environ Sci Pollut Res. 2024;31(17):25589–99. https://doi.org/10.1007/s11356-024-32821-0.

14. Zhou Q, Wei-Liang W, Lin C-Q, Liang H, Long C-Y, Lv F, Pan J-L, Liu Z-T, Wang B-Y, Yang X-F, Deng X-L, Jiang A-M. Occurrence and dietary exposure assessment of pentachlorophenol in livestock, poultry, and aquatic foods marketed in Guangdong Province, China: based on food monitoring data from 2015 to 2018. J Food Sci. 2021;86(3):1132–43. https://doi.org/10.1111/1750-3841.15653.

15. Qianyun X, Ai S, Ge G, Wang X, Li J, Gao X, Zhao S, Liu Z. Human health ambient water quality criteria and risk assessment of pentachlorophenol in Poyang Lake Basin, China. Environ Geochem Health. 2023;45:3669–82. https://doi.org/10.1007/s10653-022-01443-1.

16. Michałowicz J, Stufka-Olczyk J, Milczarek A, Michniewicz M. Analysis of annual fluctuations in the content of phenol, chlorophenols and their derivatives in chlorinated drinking waters. Environ Sci Pollut Res Int. 2011;18(7):1174–83.

17. Muir J, Eduljee G. PCP in the freshwater and marine environment of the European Union. Sci Total Environ. 1999;236(1–3):41–56.

18. Cessna AJ, Waite DT, Constable M. Concentrations of pentachlorophenol in atmospheric samples from three Canadian locations, 1994. Bull Environ Contam Toxicol. 1997;58(4):651–8.

19. Heudorf U, Letzel S, Peters M, Angerer J. PCP in the blood plasma: current exposure of the population in Germany, based on data obtained in 1998. Int J Hyg Environ Health. 2000;203(2):135–9.

20. Seifert B, Becker K, Helm D, Krause C, Schulz C, Seiwert M. The German Environmental Survey 1990/1992 (GerES II): reference concentrations of selected environmental pollutants in blood, urine, hair, house dust, drinking water and indoor air. J Expo Anal Environ Epidemiol. 2000;10(6 Pt 1):552–65.

21. Ward MH, Colt JS, Metayer C, Gunier RB, Lubin J, Crouse V, et al. Residential exposure to polychlorinated biphenyls and organochlorine pesticides and risk of childhood leukemia. Environ Health Perspect. 2009;117(6):1007–13.

22. Yan X, Zhao Q, Yan Z, Chen X, He P, Li S, Fang Y. Determination of pentachlorophenol in seafood samples from Zhejiang Province using pass-through SPE-UPLC-MS/MS: occurrence and human dietary exposure risk. Molecules. 2023;28:6394. https://doi.org/10.3390/molecules28176394.

23. Brambilla G, Fochi I, De Filippis SP, Iacovella N, di Domenico A. Pentachlorophenol, polychlorodibenzodioxin and polychlorodibenzofuran in eggs from hens exposed to contaminated wood shavings. Food Addit Contam Part A Chem Anal Control Expo Risk Assess. 2009;26(2):258–64.

24. Piskorska-Pliszczynska J, Strucinski P, Mikolajczyk S, Maszewski S, Rachubik J, Pajurek M. Pentachlorophenol from an old henhouse as a dioxin source in eggs and related human exposure. Environ Pollut. 2016;208(Pt B):404–12.

25. Zhang Y, Mhungu F, Zhang W, Wang Y, Li H, Liu Y, Li Y, Gan P, Pan X, Huang J, Zhong X, Song S, Liu Y, Chen K. Probabilistic risk assessment of dietary exposure to pentachlorophenol in Guangzhou, China. Food Addit Contam Part A. 2023;40(2):262–70. https://doi.org/10.1080/19440049.2022.2163301.

26. Pizarro C, González-Sáiz JM, Pérez-del-Notario N. Multiple response optimisation based on desirability functions of a microwave-assisted extraction method for the simultaneous determination of chloroanisoles and chlorophenols in oak barrel sawdust. J Chromatogr A. 2006;1132(1–2):8–14.
27. Ozhan D, Anli RE, Vural N, Bayram M. Determination of chloroanisoles and chlorophenols in cork and wine by using HS-SPME and GC-ECD detection. J Inst Brew. 2009;115(1):71–7.
28. Radosavljević V. Urinarni markeri ekspozicije hemijskim kancerogenima—nove smernice u preventivnoj onkologiji (Urinary markers of exposure to chemical carcinogens—new guidelines in preventive oncology). Beograd: Medija centar „Odbrana"; 2024.
29. Radosavljevic V. Urinary markers/metabolites of exposure to chemical carcinogens—new possibilities in preventive oncology. Ecotoxicol Environ Saf. 2024; https://doi.org/10.1016/j.ecoenv.2023.115774.

23.1 Overview

Polychlorinated biphenyls (PHBs) are synonymous with chlorinated biphenyls, chlorinated diphenyls and chlorobiphenyls. According to the position and number of chlorine atoms, there are 209 individual PHB compounds (congeners), of which more than 60% are tetra- and hexachlorophenyls (four and six chlorine atoms). Commercial products contain between 21% and 68% chlorine.

Twelve congeners were designated as "dioxin-like" (namely, PHB-77, PHB-81, PHB-105, PHB-114, PHB-118, PHB-123, PHB-126, PHB-156, PHB-157, PHB-167, PHB-169, and PHB-189). The activities of these PHB congeners are not only dioxin-like. At high temperatures, PHBs are flammable and as combustion products release polychlorinated dibenzofurans (PHDBFs), hydrogen chloride and polychlorinated dibenzodioxins (PHDBDs) [1, 2]. PHBs have never been used as single compounds, but as complex mixtures. Commercial PHB products consist of about 100–140 PHB congeners [3, 4].

Impurities such as 2,3,7,8-tetrachlorodibenzofuran and 2,3,4,7,8-pentachlorodib enzofuran have been reported in varying amounts in final products such as Aroclor 1248, Aroclor 1254, HLophen A-60, Phenochlor DP-6, and Kanechlor 400 [5].

23.2 Occurrence in the Environment and Exposure

PHBs are found worldwide in all parts of the environment (soil, water, air), in wildlife, and in the human body (at measurable levels). Humans are mainly exposed to PHBs through contaminated food and to a lesser extent through inhalation and dermal absorption [6–8]. PHB is absorbed by organic carbon in the soil. If absorbed, PHBs are relatively persistent [6]. In the soil, the activity of aerobic bacteria breaks down less chlorinated congeners, and anaerobic bacteria cause partial

© The Author(s), under exclusive license to Springer Nature
Switzerland AG 2025
V. Radosavljevic, *Assessing Human Exposure to Key Chemical Carcinogens*,
https://doi.org/10.1007/978-3-031-84441-6_23

dechlorination of more chlorinated congeners. PHB congener patterns in sediments change over time due to bacterial activity [10]. The patterns of PHBs found in environmental biota are called "searched," because they are the result of changes and should be taken into account during studies with experimental animals exposed to commercial PHB products.

23.2.1 Diffuse Sources of PHB in the World

PHBs have been released into the environment from many large industries in North America through inadvertent leakage, volatilization during the manufacturing process, and removal from landfills. Consequently, contamination has occurred in many rivers and streams near these sites. Many chemical plants in Western Europe are located along important rivers (Rhine, Rhone, Seine), so there have been several isolated incidents of organic chemical pollution in rivers. The Seine estuary was one of the most polluted in Europe [11]. The Venetian Lagoon in Italy is particularly polluted due to its proximity to the industrial district of Marghera Harbour [12]. In the Slovak Republic, the "Hemko" factory discharged PHB into the Laborec River, which resulted in long-term environmental contamination. During the conflict in the former Yugoslavia and the bombing in 1999, the burning or damage of industrial and military targets led to the release of large amounts of PHB into the environment. After the Kragujevac bombing, 2500 kg of PHB-based oil leaked from the Zastava Automobile industry transformer. In France in 1987 the number of installed transformers containing at least 100 kg of PHBs was 100,000 units, and in Spain in 1997 there was about 6000 tons of PHBs, although the amount of material containing or contaminated with PHBs could reach 200,000 tons [12]. In Asia, soil contamination has been reported in the Russian Federation, China, Vietnam, and Japan, either from PHB production facilities (China, Japan, Democratic People's Republic of Korea) or from e-waste recycling facilities (China) [12]. In South and Central America, the use of transformers and other devices containing PHB is widespread. There was no production of PHB in Africa, but there was widespread use of transformers and other devices containing PHB. Some studies have shown an increase in the number of PHB sources due to leakage and mis-disposal of transformers, shipwrecks, biomass burning, and the importation of e-waste and increased capacity for its recycling, usually illegal but common in Ghana, Nigeria, Kenya, the United Republic of Tanzania, South Africa, Uganda, Morocco, and Senegal [12, 13].

23.2.2 Air and Dust

Vegetation can be used as a natural passive indicator of PHB congeners. For example, pine needles reflect up to several years of exposure to PHB [14]. Tree bark integrates atmospheric concentrations of PHBs during the life of the tree [15]. Polyurethane foam was used to collect airborne PHB congeners in a confined space [16].

Outdoor Air PHB concentrations in the air depend on temperature (volatility and precipitation) and proximity to local sources (industrial facilities, landfills, and contaminated water). Combustion and other high-temperature processes generate PHBs in the air, so particulate-bound PHBs are dispersed to local and distant locations [17]. The main sources are from landfills, sewage sludge, and transformer storage [18]. There are large differences in PHB air concentrations between urban, rural, and remote locations, with the highest concentrations recorded in Toronto and the eastern USA (using passive air tracer results from 31 stations in Canada and the USA) [19]. In Europe, declining PHB concentrations have been observed since the 1960s and early 1970s—by 67% in France [20] and by 78% in the United Kingdom [21] over 20 years. Measurements in the Baltic region showed that PHB concentrations in southern Norway were higher or similar to those in urban areas. They were measured at four locations in the Czech Republic, Finland, Sweden, and the Netherlands from 1996 to 2001, but the measured values did not vary noticeably during the measurement period at any location. This suggests that a steady state has been reached between degradation and environmental cycles [22]. Very high concentrations of PHB have been reported in Senegal [23], Côte d'Ivoire, and the Gambia [24], as well as in some areas in South Africa, Kenya, Egypt, the Democratic Republic of the Congo, Ghana, Mali, and Sudan and are likely due to electronic waste landfill.

Indoor Air (Range Levels in Picograms) The main sources of PHBs indoors are sealants, paints, floor sealants, ballasts in lighting fixtures, and contaminated dust [25, 26]. PHBs can migrate into surrounding materials, such as concrete or wood, and into indoor air [27–32]. In the USA, indoor air concentrations of PHBs have been reported to be from five to 300 times higher than those in outdoor air [33] and that concentrations are higher in older buildings. In Europe, the highest indoor concentrations are found in buildings built between 1960 and 1975, sealed with elastic materials containing PHB [34–36].

23.2.3 Water

In water, PHB can be in solution or bound to particles. Inputs of PHB into the hydrological cycle are through discharge of sewage and industrial effluents, urban runoff, leachate from solid waste landfills, atmospheric deposition, and agricultural runoff [37]. In the USA, the EPA (Environmental Protection Agency) has set a goal of zero PHB in drinking water [38], but the Great Lakes of the USA and Canada are contaminated by multiple sources of PHB [39, 40], such as industrial sites on rivers [41]. The Hudson River in New York was heavily contaminated with PHBs from two large capacitor plants [42]. The Fox River in Wisconsin was heavily contaminated by copy paper manufacturers [43], and the St. Lawrence River and several of its tributaries were contaminated by the discharge of PHB-containing hydraulic fluid in drains from aluminum foundries [44]. In Europe, the highest concentrations were recorded in urban and industrial wastewater (Marseille and Barcelona) and in river discharges (from the Rhône). PHB concentrations from coastal and open waters of the western Mediterranean were of the same order of magnitude as those reported in other regions, for example, in the North Sea and North Atlantic [9]. The Danube River is the main source of contamination of the Black Sea, but many chlorinated hydrocarbons have been banned in the past decades by several European and other countries [45–47]. The areas most polluted by flood disasters are in Poland (Odra River) [48, 49]. The main source of fresh water contamination in Europe is the diffuse washing of consumer products, from households and industry into wastewater streams [50]. Industrial contamination is known to have occurred in Germany (the rivers Elbe and Rhine and their tributaries) [51], in the former Czechoslovakia (Forest Lakes) [52], in England and Ireland [53, 54], and in Slovenia through the disposal of industrial waste in Krupa river. PHB contamination also occurred in the Balkans, in Serbia (in Pančevo, Novi Sad, Belgrade, Kragujevac) after NATO's military intervention in the spring of 1999.

23.2.4 Food

Food items are regularly analyzed for PHB in various food monitoring [55, 56], and dietary studies have been conducted to identify PHB intake from food [57–59]. Eggs are usually analyzed for PHB, with a focus on yolks [57, 60]. Foods rich in lipids are more risky and analyzed more often than fruits and vegetables. Since the early 1990s, the consumption of fatty foods has been identified as a major route of exposure to PHB, PHDD, and PHDF [1, 61, 62]. PHB accumulates in edible fish, seals, and whales, and this dietary exposure has led to arctic residents to PHB concentrations that were higher than those of individuals living in temperate latitudes [63, 64]. PHBs in traditional food products are generally reduced [65]. In Africa, the primary source of PHB is dairy products, in which concentrations were several times higher than in such products in developed countries. In Europe, the main contributors to PHB for almost all groups of infants and young children appear to be milk and milk products [66, 67], and fish and seafood products for all age groups [68–70]. The Baltic Sea area is heavily contaminated with PHBs [71], which is clearly confirmed by oily fish samples from the east coast of Sweden [72]. A more comprehensive assessment of PHB concentrations in food was made by the European Agency for Food Safety (EABH) [61, 73, 74], and for the member countries of the European Union, Switzerland and Norway, in a report that included all food groups together, the range of PHB levels was in picograms and less. More than 90% of exposure to PHBs in Europe in the general population is via food consumption [69]. In China, the estimated daily intake of dioxin-like polychlorinated biphenyls (DS-PHBs) is lower than the daily intake in some developed countries [75]. Chronic exposure to PHBs can result from high consumption of fish. Fishing cohorts from the east and west coast of Sweden were established in 1965 and 1968, respectively [72]. A statistically significant increase in incidence was reported for colon cancer in the East Coast cohort. Regular consumption of predatory fish is a major source of exposure to PHBs for residents of the Great Lakes Basin [9]. Specific subpopulations have high dietary exposure to PHBs, such as Baltic Sea fishermen [70], but infant exposure to PHB6 and DL-PHB through human milk is about twice the average daily intake of adults [9].

23.3 Exposure of the General Population

Cooking oil contaminated with "canechlor" was the source of two accidental mass poisonings: in western Japan (called "Yusho," in 1968—about 1800 people) and in Taiwan, China (called "Yucheng" in 1978–1979—about 2000 people). Victims in Japan developed a "strange skin disease" as well as eye discharge and swelling of the eyelids [76–83]. Victims in China after several months developed chloracne, hyperpigmentation, severe fatigue, peripheral neuropathy, and other signs and symptoms similar to "Yusho patients." In the "Belgian dioxin crisis," 50 kg of commercial PHB mixture accidentally contaminated with 1 g of dioxin reached a supply of 500 tons of animal feed and more than 2500 poultry and pig farms were at risk. Chickens showed signs of edema [9].

23.4 Production and Use of PHB

Production peaked in the 1960s and 1970s and ceased in most countries in the late 1970s or early 1980s. Commercial products have been marketed under more than a hundred different trade names, depending on the place of production, production process, and chlorine content [9]. PHBs have been used for military purposes, but that information is usually very scarce. The predominant application of PHB was in dielectric fluids in capacitors and transformers [9]. They were used as the main ingredient in permanent elastic sealants and as flame retardant coatings [84]. Use as a plasticizer in sealants and flooring materials was common in many countries, representing up to 15–20% of total PHB use in Sweden. Sealants were mainly used in exterior applications, but indoor applications were not uncommon [85]. The use of flooring materials was limited to indoor use. Sealants analyzed about 40 years after application often contained PHB concentrations of 5–15%, in some cases as high as 35%. Some authors indicate that the inner parts of the sealant contain higher concentrations of PHB than the surface parts [86]. PHBs have also been used in inks, adhesives, microencapsulation of inks for carbonless paper, conveyor belts, rubber products, paints, pesticide fillers, plasticizers, polyoleic catalyst supports, microscope immersion oils, cutting oils, and lubricants in fluorescent surface coating lights and metal coatings [2, 87, 88]. Improper disposal of equipment containing PHBs (electronic waste) has been identified as a source of environmental pollution with PHBs, especially for old equipment [89]. Stockpiles of PHB awaiting elimination have appeared successively in many countries. The most common technology used to destroy PHBs is incineration. France has installed capacity to incinerate PHB residues for about 20,000 tons per year [90]. Water is the main route for the migration of PHBs, although PHBs are lipophilic and poorly soluble in water. Air is a less important pathway for PHB migration. PHBs are semi-volatile compounds. Less chlorinated PHB congeners have higher solubility but are more volatile than more chlorinated PHBs [91]. Airborne PHBs originate from industrial floors; military sites; contaminated water; waste sites; incineration and other forms of combustion; sewage sludge applied to agricultural land, construction materials, and paints [33]; and sealants, floor sealants, adhesives, and plasticizers in older buildings [92]. Finally, environmental PHBs enter the food chain and bioaccumulate in plants and animal fats. They are found in the fat of all meat animals, in all dairy products containing fat, and in eggs [2, 93]. PHB concentrations are usually highest in carnivorous fish from contaminated waters. Farmers often feed livestock with fishmeal or oil, or waste animal fat, leading to recycling of PHB [93]. For example, farmed salmon fed concentrated fishmeal or fish oil containing significant amounts of PHB contained elevated concentrations of PHB in adipose tissue [94]. PHBs found in food are typically more chlorinated [9]. Harad et al. suggest that inhalation may account for 15% of total human exposure to PHBs. PHBs can even be in dust indoors, especially in homes where sealant containing PHBs has been used [95]. The general public is exposed to multiple sources of PHB, very rarely a single commercial product. However, genetic differences between individuals cause differences in metabolic activity and different metabolism of congeners.

23.4.1 Occurrence in Products Other Than Commercial PHB Preparations

PHBs have been found in various paint pigments [96, 97] and electronic equipment. Since determining the presence of PHBs is a difficult process, the Basel Convention established a so-called "grey list" of materials suspected of containing PHBs: cable insulators; rubber and felt seals; thermal insulation materials including fiberglass, felt, foam, and cork; transformers; capacitors; voltage regulators; switches; bushings and electromagnets; adhesives and tapes; oil contained in electrical equipment and motors; anchor winches; hydraulic systems; surface contamination of machinery and other solid surfaces; oil-based paints; gaskets; rubber insulating supports; supports for foundations; pipe holders; light ballasts; and plasticizers [98, 99].

Mortality from cancer of the digestive tract has statistically significantly increased. Deaths from lymphoma cancer were on the rise, especially from Hodgkin's disease in women. Men were at increased risk of mortality from biliary tract cancer and prostate cancer [100]. Urinary metabolites for 2,3,4,7,8-pentachlorodibenzofuran are methoxy-pentaHDF and dimethoxy-pentachlorobiphenyl [101].

Appendix: Exposure Evaluation Questionnaire

1. During the last week, have you consumed a large amount of river fish (catfish, pike, perch) or fish from a pond? If so, when was it, how many times did you consume it, and in what quantity?..

2. During the last week, have you consumed large amounts of sea fish (salmon, tuna, herring, mackerel, anchovies, cod, etc.) or seafood (shellfish, squid, crabs)? If so, when was it, how many times did you consume it, and in what quantity?..

3. Have you worked in the paint industry? If so, in which industries, when, in which jobs, and for how long?..

4. Did you live near paint factories? If so, to which paint factories, when, at what distance, and for how long?..

5. During the last week, have you consumed a large amount of beef steak, fried chicken, beef, eggs, or French fries? If so, when was it, how many times did you consume it, and in what quantity?..

6. Have you worked in the color pigment or polymer resin industry? If so, in which industries, when, in which jobs, and for how long?..

7. Have you lived near factories of colored pigments or polymer resins? If so, to which paint factories, when, at what distance, and for how long?......................
....
....
....
....
....

8. During the last week, did you consume a large amount of milk and milk products? If so, when was it, which dairy products did you consume, how many times, and in what quantity? ....
....
....
....
....

9. Have you worked in the industry of plasticizers, building sealants, fluorescent lamps, or flame retardants? If so, in which industries, when, on what jobs, and for how long?...
....
....

10. Have you lived near factories for plasticizers, building sealants, fluorescent bulbs, or flame retardants? If so, in which paint factories, when, at what distance, and for how long?...
....
....
....
....

11. Did you work in the industry of transformers or capacitors, that is, in the production of liquids used for their cooling? If so, in which industries, when, in which jobs, and for how long?...
....
....
....

12. Did you live in the vicinity of transformer, condenser, or liquid production plants used for their cooling? If so, near which factories, when, at what distance, and for how long?...
....
....
....
....

13. Have you worked in the industry of adhesives, printer ink, insulators, paints, or pesticides? If so, in which industries, when, in which jobs, and for how long?
....
....
....
....

14. Have you lived near glue, printer ink, insulator, paint, or pesticide factories? If so, near which factories, when, at what distance, and for how long?.................
....
....
....
....
....

15. Have you worked in the recycling industry or in landfills? If so, in which industries, when, in which jobs, and for how long? ....
....
....
....
....
....

16. Have you lived near a recycling industry or a landfill? If so, near which factories or landfills, when, at what distance, and for how long?
....
....
....
....

17. Did you work in steel mills or were you exposed to burning coal or wood? If so, in which industries, when, in which jobs, and for how long? ....
....
....
....
....

18. Have you lived near a steel mill or a place with intensive burning of coal or wood? If so, near which steel mills or places with intensive burning of coal or wood, when, at what distance, and for how long? ....
....
....
....
....

19. Did you work in the ceramics industry or were you a ceramist? If so, in which industries, when, in which jobs, and for how long did you work?........................
....
....
....
....
....

20. Have you worked in the electronics industry, electronic recycling centers, or the paper industry? If so, in which industries, when, in which jobs, and how long have you been working? ....
....
....
....
....

21. Have you lived near an electronic industry, electronic recycling centers, or a paper industry? If so, near which industries, when, at what distance, and for how long? ....

22. Have you lived in buildings built between 1950 and 1970? If so, when and how long did you live in them? ....

23. Have you lived or worked in dusty conditions? If so, where, when, and how long did you live there? ....

24. Have you worked in the silicone rubber or oil industry? If so, in which industries, when, in which jobs, and for how long did you work? ....

25. Do you live in a rural, urban, or industrial region? If in an urban or industrial region, near which industries, when, at what distance, and how long did you live there? ....

26. Are there any patients with non-Hodgkin's lymphoma in your area (neighborhood or at work)? If there are, how many are there and how much time do you spend with them or in their surroundings?..

27. During the last week before the urinalysis, did you often consume fatty foods? Which one, in what quantity, and how often do you consume it? ....
....
....
....
....

28. Do you work in a rural, urban, or industrial region? If so, in an urban or industrial region, near which industries, when, at what distance, and how long did you work there? ....
....
....
....

29. Do you work with plaster or plaster? If so, in which industries, when, in which jobs, and for how long did you work? ....
....
....
....
....

30. Do you work in stores or in the production of TV/radio/stereo/video players/phones/tablets? If so, in which industries, when, in which jobs, and for how long did you work? ....
....
....
....

31. Do you work in the vehicle recycling industry? If so, in which industries, when, in which jobs, and for how long did you work?.....................
....
....
....

References

1. IPCS. Polychlorinated biphenyls and terphenyls, Environmental health criteria 140. 2nd ed. Geneva: World Health Organization, International Programme on Chemical Safety; 1993. Available from http://www.inchem.org/documents/ehc/ehc/ehc140.htm. Accessed 10 June 2014.
2. ATSDR. Toxicological profile for polychlorinated biphenyls (update). Atlanta: US Department of Health and Human Services, Public Health Service, Agency for Toxic Substances and Disease Registry; 2000. Available from http://www.atsdr.cdc.gov/ToxProfiles/tp17.pdf. Accessed 10 June 2014.

3. Frame GM, Cochran JW, Bøwadt SS. Complete PCB congener distributions for 17 Aroclor mixtures determined by 3 HRGC systems optimized for comprehensive, quantitative, congener-specific analysis. J High Resolut Chromatogr. 1996;19(12):657–68.

4. Johnson GW, Quensen JF 3rd, Chiarenzelli JR, et al. Polychlorinated biphenyls. In: Morrison RD, Murphy BL, editors. Environmental forensics: contaminant specific guide. Academic; 2000. p. 187–214.

5. de Voogt P, Brinkman UAT. Production, properties and usage of polychlorinated biphenyls. In: Kimbrough J, editor. Halogenated biphenyls, terphenyls, naphthalenes, dibenzo-dioxins and related products. Amsterdam: Elsevier Science Publishers; 1989. p. 3–43.

6. Montano L, Pironti C, Pinto G, Ricciardi M, Buono A, Brogna C, Venier M, Piscopo M, Amoresano A, Motta O. Polychlorinated biphenyls (PCBs) in the environment: occupational and exposure events, effects on human health and fertility. Toxics. 2022;10:365. https://doi.org/10.3390/toxics10070365.

7. Idowu IG, Megson D, Tiktak G, Dereviankin M, Sandau CD. Polychlorinated biphenyl (PCB) half-lives in humans: a systematic review. Chemosphere. 2023;345:140359. 140359 ISSN 0045-6535.

8. Weitekamp CA, Phillips LJ, Carlson LM, DeLuca NM, Cohen EA, Hubal GM, Lehmann. A state-of-the-science review of polychlorinated biphenyl exposures at background levels: relative contributions of exposure routes. Sci Total Environ. 2021;776 https://doi.org/10.1016/j.scitotenv.2021.145912.

9. Buckley-Golder D. Compilation of EU dioxins exposure and health data. Summary Report for European Commission DG Environment and the UK Department of the Environmental Transport and the Regions; 1999. Available from http://www.greenpeace.se/files/file_72.pdf. Accessed 23 June 2014.

10. Hardell S, Tilander H, Welfinger-Smith G, Burger J, Carpenter DO. Levels of polychlorinated biphenyls (PCBs) and three organochlorine pesticides in fish from the Aleutian Islands of Alaska. PLoS One. 2010;5(8):e12396.

11. RNO. Surveillance du Milieu Marin Travaux du Réseau National d'Observation de la qualité du milieu marin. IFREMER Edition; 2012. Available from http://envlit.ifremer.fr/documents/publications. Accessed 26 Mar 2015.

12. IARC. Polychlorinated biphenyls and polybrominated biphenyls. IARC Monogr Eval Carcinog Risks Hum. 2016;107:1–510.

13. UNEP. Sustainable innovation and technology transfer industrial sector studies: recycling—from E-waste to resources. United Nations Environment Programme; 2009. Available from http://www.unep.org/pdf/Recycling_From_e-waste_to_resources.pdf. Accessed 24 June 2014.

14. Kylin H. Airborne lipophilic pollutants in pine needles. Doctoral dissertation. Environmental chemistry. Stockholm: Wallenberg Laboratory Stockholm University; 1994.

15. Hermanson MH, Hites RA. Polychlorinated biphenyls in tree bark. Environ Sci Technol. 1990;24(5):666–71.

16. Hazrati S, Harrad S. Causes of variability in concentrations of polychlorinated biphenyls and polybrominated diphenyl ethers in indoor air. Environ Sci Technol. 2006;40(24):7584–9.

17. Othman N, Ismail Z, Selamat MI, Sheikh Abdul Kadir SH, Shibraumalisi NA. A review of polychlorinated biphenyls (PCBs) pollution in the air: where and how much are we exposed to? Int J Environ Res Public Health. 2022;19:13923. https://doi.org/10.3390/ijerph192113923.

18. Hsu YK, Holsen TM, Hopke PK. Locating and quantifying PCB sources in Chicago: receptor modeling and field sampling. Environ Sci Technol. 2003;37(4):681–90.

19. Shen L, Wania F, Lei YD, Teixeira C, Muir DC, Xiao H. Polychlorinated biphenyls and polybrominated diphenyl ethers in the North American atmosphere. Environ Pollut. 2006;144(2):434–44.

20. EC. Dioxins & PCBs: environmental levels and human exposure in candidate countries. European Commission Final Report ENV.C.2/SER/2002/0085; 2004.

21. CITEPA. Polychlorinated biphenyls—PCB. Paris: Centre Interprofessionnel Technique d'Etudes de la Pollution Atmosphérique; 2013. Available from http://www.citepa.org/fr/air-et-climat/polluants/polluantorganiques-persistants/polychlorobiphenyls. Accessed 24 June 2014.

22. Holoubek I, Brörström-Lundén E, Duyzer J, Shatalov V, Klánová J. Regional trends of POPs in European ambient air. Brno: Masaryk University; 2003. Available from http://www.recetox.muni.cz/coe/sources/workshop_1_rba_pts/VI08Holoubek2.pdf. accessed 24 June 2014.

23. Klánová J, Cupr P, Holoubek I, Borůvková J, Pribylová P, Kares R, et al. Monitoring of persistent organic pollutants in Africa. Part 1: passive air sampling across the continent in 2008. J Environ Monit. 2009;11(11):1952–63.

24. Gioia R, Eckhardt S, Breivik K, Jaward FM, Prieto A, Nizzetto L, et al. Evidence for major emissions of PCBs in the West African region. Environ Sci Technol. 2011;45(4):1349–55.

25. Rayhan MRI, Akbor A, Nahar A, Chowdhury NJ, Mostafizur Rahman AHM, Saadat. Exposure of polychlorinated biphenyls *via* indoor dust particles and their health risks in Dhaka City, Bangladesh. J Hazard Mater Adv. 2024;14:100421. https://doi.org/10.1016/j.hazadv.2024.100421.

26. Hammel SC, Andersen HV, Knudsen LE, Frederiksen M. Inhalation and dermal absorption as dominant pathways of PCB exposure for residents of contaminated apartment buildings. Int J Hyg Environ Health. 2023;247:114056. https://doi.org/10.1016/j.ijheh.2022.114056.

27. Vorhees DJ, Cullen AC, Altshul LM. Exposure to polychlorinated biphenyls in residential indoor air and outdoor air near a superfund site. Environ Sci Technol. 1997;31(12):3612–8.

28. Vorhees DJ, Cullen AC, Altshul LM. Polychlorinated biphenyls in house dust and yard soil near a superfund site. Environ Sci Technol. 1999;33(13):2151–6.

29. Herrick RF, McClean MD, Meeker JD, Baxter LK, Weymouth GA. An unrecognized source of PCB contamination in schools and other buildings. Environ Health Perspect. 2004;112(10):1051–3.

30. Colt JS, Severson RK, Lubin J, Rothman N, Camann D, Davis S, et al. Organochlorines in carpet dust and non-Hodgkin lymphoma. Epidemiology. 2005;16(4):516–25.

31. Franzblau A, Zwica L, Knutson K, Chen Q, Lee SY, Hong B, et al. An investigation of homes with high concentrations of PCDDs, PCDFs, and/or dioxin-like PCBs in house dust. J Occup Environ Hyg. 2009;6(3):188–99.

32. Harrad S, Ibarra C, Robson M, Melymuk L, Zhang X, Diamond M, et al. Polychlorinated biphenyls in domestic dust from Canada, New Zealand, United Kingdom and United States: implications for human exposure. Chemosphere. 2009;76(2):232–8.

33. Wallace JC, Basu I, Hites RA. Sampling and analysis artifacts caused by elevated indoor air polychlorinated biphenyl concentrations. Environ Sci Technol. 1996;30(9):2730–4.

34. Balfanz E, Fuchs J, Kieper H. Sampling and analysis of polychlorinated biphenyls (PCB) in indoor air due to permanently elastic sealants. Chemosphere. 1993;26(5):871–80.

35. Kohler M, Tremp J, Zennegg M, Seiler C, Minder-Kohler S, Beck M, et al. Joint sealants: an overlooked diffuse source of polychlorinated biphenyls in buildings. Environ Sci Technol. 2005;39(7):1967–73.

36. Wilkins K, Bøwadt S, Larsen K, Sporring S. Detection of indoor PCB contamination by thermal desorption of dust. A rapid screening method? Environ Sci Pollut Res Int. 2002;9(3):166–8.

37. Scrimshaw MD, Bubb JM, Lester JN. Organochlorine contamination of UK Essex coast salt marsh sediments. J Coast Res. 1996;12:246–55.

38. EPA. Basic information about polychlorinated biphenyls (PCBs) in drinking water. United States Environmental Protection Agency; 2014. Available from http://water.epa.gov/drink/contaminants/basicinformation/polychlorinated-biphenyls.cfm. Accessed 11 May 2015.

39. Bhavsar SP, Jackson DA, Hayton A, Reiner EJ, Chen T, Bodnar J. Are PCB levels in fish from Canadian Great Lakes still declining? J Great Lakes Res. 2007;33(3):592–605.

40. Turyk ME, Bhavsar SP, Bowerman W, Boysen E, Clark M, Diamond M, et al. Risks and benefits of consumption of Great Lakes fish. Environ Health Perspect. 2012;120(1):11–8.

41. Kelly TH, Czuczwa JM, Sticksel PR, Sverdrup GM, Koval PJ, Hodanbosi RF. Atmospheric and tributary inputs of toxic substances to Lake Erie. J Great Lakes Res. 1991;17(4):504–16.
42. Carpenter DO, Welfinger-Smith G. The Hudson River: a case study of PCB contamination. In: Selendy JMH, editor. Water and sanitation-related diseases and the environment. Hoboken: Wiley-Blackwell; 2011. p. 303–27.
43. Imamoglu I, Li K, Christensen ER, McMullin JK. Sources and dechlorination of polychlorinated biphenyl congeners in the sediments of Fox River, Wisconsin. Environ Sci Technol. 2004;38(9):2574–83.
44. Fitzgerald EF, Brix KA, Deres DA, Hwang SA, Bush B, Lambert G, et al. Polychlorinated biphenyl (PCB) and dichlorodiphenyl dichloroethylene (DDE) exposure among Native American men from contaminated Great Lakes fish and wildlife. Toxicol Ind Health. 1996;12(3–4):361–8.
45. Winkels HJ, Kroonenberg SB, Lychagin MY, Marin G, Rusakov GV, Kasimov NS. Geochronology of priority pollutants in sedimentation zones of the Volga and Danube delta in comparison with the Rhine delta. Appl Geochem. 1998;13(5):581–91.
46. Covaci A, Gheorghe A, Hulea O, Schepens P. Levels of organochlorinated pollutants (PCBs, OCPs and PBDEs) in biota from the Danube Delta, Romania. Organohalogen Compd. 2002;59:9–12.
47. Fillmann G, Readman JW, Tolosa I, Bartocci J, Villeneuve JP, Cattini C, et al. Persistent organochlorine residues in sediments from the Black Sea. Mar Pollut Bull. 2002;44(2):122–33.
48. Wolska L, Wardencki W, Wiergowski M, Zygmunt B, Zabiegała B, Konieczka P, et al. Evaluation of pollution degree of the Odra River basin with organic compounds after the 1997 summer flood—general comments. Acta Hydrochim Hydrobiol. 1999;27(5):343–9.
49. Protasowicki M, Niedźwiecki E, Ciereszko W, et al. The comparison of sediment contamination in the area of estuary and the lower course of the Odra before and after the flood of summer 1997. Acta Hydrochim Hydrobiol. 1999;27:338–42.
50. UNEP. Mediterranean regional report: regionally based assessment of persistent toxic substances. Global Environment Facility, United Nations Environment Programme Chemicals; 2002. Available from http://www.unep.org/chemicalsandwaste/. Accessed 24 June 2014.
51. Brauch HJ. Pesticides in the River Rhine. Acta Hydrochim Hydrobiol. 1993;21(3):137–44.
52. Nondek L, Frolikova N. Polychlorinated biphenyls in the hydrosphere of Czechoslovakia. Chemosphere. 1991;23(3):269–80.
53. Sanders G, Jones J, Hamilton-Taylor J, Doerr H. Historical inputs of polychlorinated biphenyls and other organochlorines to a dated lacustrine sediment core in rural England. Environ Sci Technol. 1992;26(9):1815–21.
54. Harrad SJ, Sewart AP, Alcock R, Boumphrey R, Burnett V, Duarte-Davidson R, et al. Polychlorinated biphenyls (PCBs) in the British environment: sinks, sources and temporal trends. Environ Pollut. 1994;85(2):131–46.
55. Fromberg A, Granby K, Højgård A, Fagt S, Larsen JC, et al. Estimation of dietary intake of PCB and organochlorine pesticides for children and adults. Food Chem. 2011;125(4):1179–87.
56. EFSA. Opinion of the scientific panel on contaminants in the food chain on a request from the Commission related to the presence of non-dioxin-like polychlorinated biphenyls (PCB) in feed and food. EFSA J. 2005;284:1–137. Available from http://www.efsa.europa.eu/en/efsajournal/doc/284.pdf. Accessed 10 June 2014.
57. Voorspoels S, Covaci A, Neels H. Dietary PCB intake in Belgium. Environ Toxicol Pharmacol. 2008;25(2):179–82.
58. Fromme H, Albrecht M, Boehmer S, Büchner K, Mayer R, Liebl B, et al. Intake and body burden of dioxin-like compounds in Germany: the INES study. Chemosphere. 2009;76(11):1457–63.
59. Saktrakulkla P, Lan T, Hua J, Marek RF, Thorne PS, Hornbuckle KC. PCBs in food. Environ Sci Technol. 2020;54(18):11443–52. https://doi.org/10.1021/acs.est.0c03632.
60. Kiviranta H, Ovaskainen ML, Vartiainen T. Market basket study on dietary intake of PCDD/Fs, PCBs, and PBDEs in Finland. Environ Int. 2004;30(7):923–32.

61. Lindell B. The nordic expert group for criteria documentation of health risks from chemicals. 146. Polychlorinated biphenyls (PCBs). Gothenburg: University of Gothenburg; 2012. ISBN 978-91-85971-35-0, ISSN 0346-7821. Available from http://www.av.se/arkiv/neg/publications/. Accessed 10 June 2014.

62. Dewailly E, Ayotte P, Bruneau S, Laliberté C, Muir DC, Norstrom RJ. Inuit exposure to organochlorines through the aquatic food chain in arctic québec. Environ Health Perspect. 1993;101(7):618–20.

63. Rigét F, Bignert A, Braune B, Stow J, Wilson S. Temporal trends of legacy POPs in Arctic biota, an update. Sci Total Environ. 2010;408(15):2874–84.

64. Huang T, Ling Z, Ma J, Macdonald RW, Gao H, Tao S, Tian C, Song S, Jiang W, Chen L, Chen K, Xie Z, Zhao Y, Zhao L, Chen G, Mao X. Human exposure to polychlorinated biphenyls embodied in global fish trade. Nat Food. 2020; https://doi.org/10.1038/s43016-020-0066-1.https.

65. Barr DB, Weihe P, Davis MD, Needham LL, Grandjean P. Serum polychlorinated biphenyl and organochlorine insecticide concentrations in a Faroese birth cohort. Chemosphere. 2006;62(7):1167–82.

66. Becker K, Göen T, Seiwert M, Conrad A, Pick-Fuss H, Müller J, et al. GerES IV: phthalate metabolites and bisphenol A in urine of German children. Int J Hyg Environ Health. 2009;212(6):685–92.

67. Langer P, Kocan A, Tajtaková M, Petrík J, Chovancová J, Drobná B, et al. Fish from industrially polluted freshwater as the main source of organochlorinated pollutants and increased frequency of thyroid disorders and dysglycemia. Chemosphere. 2007;67(9):S379–85.

68. Fréry N, Volatier JL, Zeghnoun A, et al. National study on serum dioxins and PCB levels in the population living around municipal solid waste incinerators (MSWI), Rapport d'étude. Saint-Maurice: French Institute for Public Health Surveillance; 2009. Available from http://opac.invs.sante.fr/index.php?lvl=notice_display&id=1031. Accessed 24 June 2014.

69. ANSES. National study on ingestion of polychlorinated biphenyls by consumers of freshwater fish, Rapport d'étude scientifique. Agence nationale de sécurité sanitaire, alimentation, environnement, travail; 2011.

70. Kiviranta H, Vartiainen T, Parmanne R, Hallikainen A, Koistinen J. PCDD/Fs and PCBs in Baltic herring during the 1990s. Chemosphere. 2003;50(9):1201–16.

71. Svensson BG, Nilsson A, Jonsson E, Schütz A, Akesson B, Hagmar L. Fish consumption and exposure to persistent organochlorine compounds, mercury, selenium and methylamines among Swedish fishermen. Scand J Work Environ Health. 1995;21(2):96–105.

72. EFSA. Results of the monitoring of dioxin levels in food and feed. EFSA J. 2010;8(3):1385. https://doi.org/10.2903/j.efsa.2010.1385. Available from www.efsa.europa.eu. Accessed 23 June 2014.

73. EFSA. Update of the monitoring of dioxins and PCBs levels in food and feed. EFSA J. 2012;10(7):2832. https://doi.org/10.2903/j.efsa.2012.2832. Available from www.efsa.europa.eu/efsajournal/doc/2832.pdf. Accessed 23 June 2014.

74. Liu G, Zheng M, Jiang G, Cai Z, Wu Y. Dioxin analysis in China. Trends Anal Chem. 2013;46:178–88.

75. Masuda Y. The Yusho rice oil poisoning incident. In: Schecter A, editor. Dioxins and health. New York: Plenum Press; 1994. p. 633–59.

76. Masuda Y, Schecter A, Päpke O. Concentrations of PCBs, PCDFs and PCDDs in the blood of Yusho patients and their toxic equivalent contribution. Chemosphere. 1998;37(9–12):1773–80.

77. Matsueda T, Iida T, Hirakawa H, Fukamachi K, Tokiwa H, Nagayama J. Toxic evaluation of PCDDs, PCDFs and coplanar PCBs in breast-fed babies of Yusho and healthy mothers. Chemosphere. 1993;27(1–3):187–94.

78. Kuratsune M. Investigation of the cause of the "strange disease". In: Kuratsune M, Yoshimura H, Hori Y, Okumura M, Masuda Y, editors. Yusho: a human disaster caused by PCBs and related compounds. Fukuoka: Kyushu University Press; 1996. p. 15–46.

79. Nagayama J, Masuda Y, Kuratsune M. Determination of polychlorinated dibenzofurans in tissues of patients with "Yusho". Food Cosmet Toxicol. 1977;15(3):195–8.

80. Tanabe S, Kannan N, Wakimoto T, Tatsukawa R, Okamoto T, Masuda Y. Isomer-specific determination and toxic evaluation of potentially hazardous coplanar PCBs, dibenzofurans and dioxins in the tissues of "Yusho" and PCB poisoning victim and in the causal oil. Toxicol Environ Chem. 1989;24(4):215–31.
81. Todaka T, Hirakawa H, Hori T, Tobiishi K, Iida T, Furue M. Concentrations of polychlorinated dibenzo-p-dioxins, polychlorinated dibenzofurans, and non-ortho and mono-ortho polychlorinated biphenyls in blood of Yusho patients. Chemosphere. 2007;66(10):1983–9.
82. Ohta S, Nakao T, Aozasa O, et al. Determination of co-planar PXBs in human breast milk from 20 women in Japan. Organohalogen Compd. 2008a;70:2207–10.
83. Heinzow B, Mohr S, Ostendorp G, Kerst M, Körner W. PCB and dioxin-like PCB in indoor air of public buildings contaminated with different PCB sources-deriving toxicity equivalent concentrations from standard PCB congeners. Chemosphere. 2007;67(9):1746–53.
84. Jansson B, Sandberg J, Johansson N, Åstebro A. PCB in elastic sealants—a major or minor problem? Swedish Environmental Agency Report 4697; 1997. [In Swedish with English summary].
85. Johansson N, Hanberg A, Wingfors H, et al. PCB in building sealant is influencing PCB levels in blood of residents. Organohalogen Compd. 2003;63:381–4.
86. Erickson MD. Introduction to PCB properties, uses, occurrence and regulatory history. In: Robertson LW, Hansen LG, editors. PCBs, recent advances in environmental toxicology and health effects. The University Press of Kentucky; 2001. ISBN 0-8131-2226-0.
87. Erickson MD, Kaley RG 2nd. Applications of polychlorinated biphenyls. Environ Sci Pollut Res Int. 2011;18(2):135–51.
88. Leung A, Cai ZW, Wong MH. Environmental contamination from electronic waste recycling at Guiyu, Southeast China. J Mater Cycle Waste Manag. 2006;8(1):21–33.
89. INERIS. State of the art of the contamination processes of equipment containing PCBs, and techniques used to control emissions thereof, No. DRC-13-133121-03381A. Ministry of Ecology, Development and Energy—General Office of Risk Prevention—Bureau of Prospective, Evaluation and Data; 2013. p. 1–75.
90. Totten LA, Stenchikov G, Gigliotti CL, Lahoti N, Eisenreich SJ. Measurement and modelling of urban atmospheric PCB concentrations on a small (8 km) spatial scale. Atmos Environ. 2006;40(40):7940–52.
91. Hu D, Hornbuckle KC. Inadvertent polychlorinated biphenyls in commercial paint pigments. Environ Sci Technol. 2010;44(8):2822–7.
92. IOM; Institute of Medicine. Dioxins and dioxin-like compounds in the food supply. Washington, DC: The National Academies Press; 2003.
93. Hites RA, Foran JA, Carpenter DO, Hamilton MC, Knuth BA, Schwager SJ. Global assessment of organic contaminants in farmed salmon. Science. 2004;303(5655):226–9.
94. Harrad S, Hazrati S, Ibarra C. Concentrations of polychlorinated biphenyls in indoor air and polybrominated diphenyl ethers in indoor air and dust in Birmingham, United Kingdom: implications for human exposure. Environ Sci Technol. 2006;40(15):4633–8.
95. Kuusisto S, Lindroos O, Rantio T, et al. Occurrence of PCB-containing indoor paints in Finland—preliminary inventory. In: de Oliveira Fernandes E, Gameiro da Silva M, Rosado Pinto J, editors. HB 2006 healthy buildings Lisboa, 4–8 June 2006. Proceedings vol. IV materials, systems and technologies for healthy buildings; 2006. p. 121–4.
96. Basel Convention. Technical guideline for the environmentally sound management of the full and partial dismantling of ships. United Nations Environment Program; 2003. Available from   http://www.basel.int/Portals/4/Basel%20Convention/docs/meetings/sbc/workdoc/techgships-e.pdf. Accessed 23 June 2014.
97. Brown DP, Jones M. Mortality and industrial hygiene study of workers exposed to polychlorinated biphenyls. Arch Environ Health. 1981;36(3):120–9.
98. Bertazzi PA, Riboldi L, Pesatori A, Radice L, Zocchetti C. Cancer mortality of capacitor manufacturing workers. Am J Ind Med. 1987;11(2):165–76.

99. Rengelshausen J, Randerath I, Schettgen T, Esser A, Kaifie A, Lang J, Kraus T, Ziegler P. Ten years after: findings from the medical surveillance program on Health Effects in High-Level Exposure to PCB (HELPcB). Arch Toxicol. 2023;97:2609–23. https://doi.org/10.1007/s00204-023-03578-1.

100. Radosavljević V. Urinarni markeri ekspozicije hemijskim kancerogenima—nove smernice u preventivnoj onkologiji (Urinary markers of exposure to chemical carcinogens—new guidelines in preventive oncology). Beograd: Medija centar „Odbrana"; 2024.

101. Radosavljevic V. Urinary markers/metabolites of exposure to chemical carcinogens—new possibilities in preventive oncology. Ecotoxicol Environ Saf. 2024; https://doi.org/10.1016/j.ecoenv.2023.115774.

Human Exposure to Polycyclic Aromatic Hydrocarbons (Shale Oil)

24

24.1 Overview

24.1.1 Occurrence in the Environment

Oil shales are sedimentary rocks that mainly contain mineral components and organic matter called kerogen. Crude oil from shale is a product of thermal processing of crude oil shale. Oil shale has a low boiling point and produces liquid organic products (oils) during thermal decomposition. Shale crude oils have a higher concentration of organic nitrogen compounds and arsenic than crude oil. They are viscous, waxy liquids consisting of hydrocarbons (alkanes, alkenes, and aromatic compounds) and polar components (organic compounds of nitrogen, oxygen, and sulfur) [1]. In order to obtain oil from shale, its organic part (kerogen) must be thermally decomposed. This process, known as retorting, converts the solid organic material (shale) into liquid and gaseous fractions and a solid carbonaceous residue. The liquid fraction, the so-called shale oil, consists of condensable hydrocarbons and small amounts of water. The gas product is a mixture of carbon monoxide, carbon dioxide, hydrogen, nitrogen, hydrogen sulfide, methane, and other hydrocarbons. Carbonaceous residue, a coke-like material, is a mixture with the inorganic minerals of the original oil shale [2].

Oil shale is found in many parts of the world, and the world's total recoverable resources are estimated at 2.6 trillion barrels [3]. They have been used in the production of fuel oil for gas turbines, automobile gasoline, and additives for petroleum fuel oil with a high sulfur content [4, 5]. In the People's Republic of China, shale oil has been used as raw material for refineries and for electricity generation [6]. They can also be used to produce gasoline, kerosene, diesel fuel, and coke [7, 8]. Oil shale industries operate in Europe (Estonia), South America (Brazil), and Asia (China).

© The Author(s), under exclusive license to Springer Nature Switzerland AG 2025
V. Radosavljevic, *Assessing Human Exposure to Key Chemical Carcinogens*,
https://doi.org/10.1007/978-3-031-84441-6_24

The largest use is in Estonia—in northeastern Estonia, about 85% of this material is burned as fuel in electric power plants, and the rest is returned for shale oil and used for the production of fuel and petrochemical products [1].

Exposure to shale oil cause malignant and nonmalignant diseases [9–13]. It is causally linked to skin cancer, especially scrotal cancer [13, 14]. 1-Hydroxypyrene is the most representative urinary metabolite from shale oils [15].

Appendix: Exposure Evaluation Questionnaire

1. Have you worked in the extraction and/or processing of oil shale? If so, what jobs did you work and for how long? ....
   ....

   ....

   ....

2. Did you live near a place where oil shale was extracted? If so, how long did you live near such a place and how far was the place where you lived from the place where the oil shale was extracted? ....
   ....

   ....

   ....

   ....

   ....

3. Have you worked on wastewater treatment from the oil shale industry? If so, what jobs did you work for and for how long?
   ....

   ....

4. Have you consumed food produced in the territory where oil (oil) shale was once extracted and/or processed (specify when)? If so, how long have you consumed it and which food? ....
   ....

   ....

   ....

   ....

   ....

5. Have you worked on the removal of waste rock (material) from the oil shale industry? If so, what jobs did you work for and for how long?
   ....

   ....

   ....

   ....

6. Did you live near a place where waste material from the oil shale industry was disposed of? If so, how long have you lived near such a place and how far was the place where you lived from where the waste material from the oil shale industry was disposed of? ....
....
....
....
....

7. Have you consumed food produced in the territory where tailings from the oil shale industry were once (specify when) disposed of? If so, how long have you consumed it and which food?...
....
....
....
....
....

8. Did you work on oil extraction and/or processing? If so, what jobs did you work and for how long? ....
....
....
....

9. Did you live near a place where oil was extracted? If so, how long did you live near such a place and how far was the place where you lived from the place where the oil was extracted? ....
....
....
....
....
....

10. Have you worked on the purification of waste water from the oil industry? If so, what jobs did you work for and for how long? ....
....
....

11. Have you consumed food produced in the territory where oil extraction and/or processing was once (specify when) carried out? If so, how long have you consumed it and which food?..
....
....
....
....
....

12. Have you worked on the removal of waste materials from the oil industry? If so, what jobs did you work for and for how long? ....
....
....
....
....

13. Have you lived near a place where waste material from the oil industry was disposed of? If so, how long have you lived near such a place and how far was the place where you lived from the place where waste material from the oil industry was disposed of? ....

14. Have you consumed food produced in the territory where once (specify when) waste material from the oil industry was dumped? If so, how long have you consumed it and which food?...

15. Did you work on extracting and/or processing natural gas? If so, what jobs did you work and for how long? ....

16. Did you live near a place where natural gas was extracted and/or processed? If so, how long have you lived near such a place and how far was the place where you lived from where natural gas was extracted and/or processed? ....

17. Have you worked on wastewater treatment from the natural gas industry? If so, what jobs did you work for and for how long? ....

18. Have you consumed food produced in the territory where extraction and/or processing of natural gas was once (specify when) performed? If so, how long have you consumed it and which food?...

19. Have you worked on the removal of waste materials from the natural gas industry? If so, what jobs did you work for and for how long? ....

....

....

....

....

20. Have you lived near a site where waste material from the natural gas industry was disposed of? If so, how long have you lived near such a place and how far was the place where you lived from the place where waste material from the natural gas industry was disposed of?..

....

....

....

....

....

21. Have you consumed food produced in the territory where waste material from the natural gas industry was once (specify when) disposed of? If so, how long have you consumed it and which food?...

....

....

....

....

....

22. Have you used water whose source is located or transported through oil shale deposits or oil shale processing industry, coal deposits or coal processing industry, oil deposits or oil processing industry, natural gas deposits, or industry natural gas processing? If so, when and for how long?...

....

....

....

References

1. IARC. Chemical agents and related occupations. IARC Monogr Eval Carcinog Risks Hum. 2012;100F:1–628.
2. Weiss HJ. Oil shale. In: Ullmann's encyclopedia of industrial chemistry. 7th ed. Weinheim: Wiley-VCH Verlag GmbH & Co. KGaA; 2005. [Online].
3. AAPG. Energy minerals division: technical area: oil shale. American Association of Petroleum Geologists; 2009. http://emd.aapg.org/technical_areas/oil_shale.cfm
4. Aarna A. Chemical engineering in the Estonian SSR. Tallinn: Perioodika; 1978. p. 29–34.
5. Öpik I, Kaganovich I. Oil shale of the Baltic basin: power engineering and thermal processing. In: Golden CO, editor. Proceedings of the 6th IIASA resources conference, world oil-shale resources and their potential development. Laxenburg: International Institute For Applied Systems Analysis; 1981.

6. Dickson PF. Oil shale. In: Kirk RE, Othmer DF, editors. Kirk-Othmer encyclopedia of chemical technology, vol. 16. 3rd ed. New York: Wiley; 1981. p. 333–57.

7. Qian JL. Oil shale industry of China. In: Synfuels' 2nd world-wide symposium. New York: McGraw-Hill; 1982. p. 1–12.

8. IARC. Polynuclear aromatic compounds, Part 4, bitumens, coal-tars and derived products, shale-oils and soots. IARC Monogr Eval Carcinog Risk Chem Hum. 1985;35:1–247.

9. Wang C-q, Ying Y, Mei X-d, Chen Z, Feng-lin X. Human health risk assessment of volatile organic compounds in oil-based drill cuttings of shale gas. Environ Sci Pollut Res. 2024;31:16092–105. https://doi.org/10.1007/s11356-024-32322-0.

10. Liu Z, Zheng T, Chen Q, Chen X, Xie Y, Wang Y, Ren M, Gao Z-q, Lin B, Feng X. Identification and health risk evaluation of soil contaminated by polycyclic aromatic hydrocarbons at shale gas extraction sites based on positive matrix factorization. Chemosphere. 2024;356:141962. https://doi.org/10.1016/j.chemosphere.2024.141962.

11. Chen K, Wu F, Liang L, Zhang K, Huang J, Cheng F, Yu Z, Hicks AL, You J. Prioritizing organic pollutants for shale gas exploitation: life cycle environmental risk assessments in China and the US. Environ Sci Technol. 2024;58(19):8149–60. https://doi.org/10.1021/acs.est.3c10288.

12. Orru H, Viitak A, Herodes K, Veber T, Lukk M. Human biomonitoring in the oil shale industry area in Estonia—overview of earlier programmes and future perspectives. Front Public Health. 2020;8:582114. https://doi.org/10.3389/fpubh.2020.582114.

13. Jameson CW. Chapter 7: polycyclic aromatic hydrocarbons and associated occupational exposures. In: Baan RA, Stewart BW, Straif K, editors. Tumour site concordance and mechanisms of carcinogenesis. Lyon: International Agency for Research on Cancer; 2019.

14. Radosavljević V. Urinarni markeri ekspozicije hemijskim kancerogenima—nove smernice u preventivnoj onkologiji (Urinary markers of exposure to chemical carcinogens—new guidelines in preventive oncology). Beograd: Medija centar „Odbrana"; 2024.

15. Radosavljevic V. Urinary markers/metabolites of exposure to chemical carcinogens—new possibilities in preventive oncology. Ecotoxicol Environ Saf. 2024; https://doi.org/10.1016/j.ecoenv.2023.115774.

25.1 Overview

25.1.1 Exposure of the General Population

Soot is a by-product of burning organic matter, such as coal, wood, fuel oil, waste oil, paper, plastic, and household waste. The chemical composition of soot is very variable (it depends on the type of burned material and combustion conditions) [1, 2]. Chemical analyses of the soot extract identified about 20 PAHs (polycyclic aromatic hydrocarbons—benz[a]anthracene, benzo[c]phenanthrene, benzo[a]pyrene, dibenz[a,h]anthracene, chryzen, indeno[1,2,3-cd]pyrene, etc.) [3], which may contribute to the genotoxic and carcinogenic activities of carbon black [4, 5]. The modern way of life, especially urbanization, favors the emergence of PAHs [6–12].

Exposure to soot gives a statistically significant increase in the number of lung, esophagus, pharynx, bladder, and colon cancers [13, 14]. 1-Hydroxypyrene is the most representative urinary metabolite from soot [15].

Appendix: Exposure Evaluation Questionnaire

1. Do you work or live in an environment with a significant presence of soot? If so, how much time do you spend daily in such an environment and how long have you lived like that?..
....
....

V. Radosavljevic, *Assessing Human Exposure to Key Chemical Carcinogens*, https://doi.org/10.1007/978-3-031-84441-6_25

2. Do you work or live in a dusty environment? If so, how much time do you spend daily in such an environment and how long have you lived like that? ....
....
....
....

3. Do you work in the industry of sintering (consolidation by heating) of ores and metals? If so, in what jobs and for how long? ....
....
....
....

4. Is there a significant number of individual fireplaces in your neighborhood and what materials are used to heat them?..
....
....
....

5. Are you exposed to burning candles? If so, when and for how long?
....
....

6. Do you work in construction? If so, in what jobs and for how long?..................
....
....
....

7. Are you exposed to soot in any way (inhalation, ingestion, through the skin) and for how long? ....
....
....
....
....
....

8. Have you been near an open fire (burning stubble in a field, forest fires)? If so, when and for how long?..
....
....
....

9. Do you work or live near a waste incinerator and for how long? ....
....
....
....
....

10. Do you work or live near a mine or quarry and for how long? ....
....
....

11. Do you work or live near major (frequent) roads and for how long? ....
....
....
....
....

12. Do you work or live near large factory chimneys? If so, how far and for how long? ....
....
....
....

13. Are you a smoker and for how long?...
....

14. Do you work as a chimney sweep and for how long? ....

15. Do you heat with a stove using wood, coal, oil, pellets, or biomass? If so, for how long (at home and at work)? ....
....
....
....

16. Are you exposed to tobacco smoke at home or at work and for how long (during the day and in total)? ....
....
....
....

17. Where do you live and work: in an urban, rural, or semi-urban environment? For how long? .....
....
....
....

18. Are you exposed to exhaust gases from motor vehicles or trains? If so, how many days and for how long? ....
....
....

19. Have you recently (when and how much) consumed charred food?...................
....
....
....

20. Are you a griller or do you often grill food (how often)?..........................
....
....

21. Do you work as a firefighter? If you work, when was the last time you were exposed to fire or smoke and for how long? ....
....
....
....

22. Have you recently been exposed to a fire (forest fire, city fire)? If so, when and for how long? ....
....
....

23. Have you consumed grilled, smoked, or fried food in the last 2 days? If so, when and how much? ....
....
....

24. Do you work or live near the industry: cement, bitumen, car tires, asphalt, petrochemical, or coke? If you work, how long have you been working and what jobs? If you live near the mentioned industries, how long have you lived there and at what distance from them?..
....
....
....
....
....

25. Do you consume food produced within a radius of 15 km from the mentioned industries? If so, when was the last time you consumed it, which food, and in what quantity? ....
....
....
....
....

26. Do you work as a car mechanic? If so, when and for how long?
....
....

27. Do you work with lubricants or as a professional driver? If so, when and for how long?...
....
....
....

28. Do you work in the railways? If so, in what jobs and for how long? .....
....
....

References

1. Zhang Z, Jingyi H, Zhang D, Jia G, Bin Zhang S, Wang WZ, Zhao Z, Zhang J. Overview of the impact of oxygenated biofuel additives on soot emissions in laboratory scale. Fuel Process Technol. 2024;254:108046. https://doi.org/10.1016/j.fuproc.2024.108046.
2. Leroy-Cancellieri V, Cancellieri D, Leoni E. Characterization of PAHs trapped in the soot from the combustion of various Mediterranean species. Atmosphere. 2021;12:965. https://doi.org/10.3390/atmos12080965.
3. IARC. Chemical agents and related occupations. IARC Monogr Eval Carcinog Risks Hum. 2012;100F:1–628.

4. Teixeira J, Bessa MJ, Delerue-Matos C, Sarmento B, Santos-Silva A, Rodrigues F, Oliveira M. Firefighters' personal exposure to gaseous PAHs during controlled forest fires: a case study with estimation of respiratory health risks and *in vitro* toxicity. Sci Total Environ. 2024;908:168364. https://doi.org/10.1016/j.scitotenv.2023.168364.

5. Moazami TN, Jørgensen RB, Svendsen KH, Teigen KA, Hegseth MN. Personal exposure to gaseous and particulate phase polycyclic aromatic hydrocarbons (PAHs) and nanoparticles and lung deposited surface area (LDSA) for soot among Norwegian chimney sweepers. J Occup Environ Hyg. 2024;21(1):24–34. https://doi.org/10.1080/15459624.2023.2264349.

6. Radosavljevic V. Environmental health and bioterrorism. In: Nriagu JO, editor. Encyclopedia of environmental health, vol. 2. 2nd ed. Burlington: Elsevier; 2019. p. 450–7.

7. Pavanello S, Genova A, Foa V, Clonfero E. Assessment of occupational exposure to aromatic polycyclic hydrocarbons determining urinary levels of 1-pyrenol. Med Lav. 2000;91:192–205.

8. Kambi M, Osuji LC, Onojake MC. Compositional pattern and human exposure risk of polycyclic aromatic hydrocarbons (PAHs) in fine dust from indoor environments in Port Harcourt, Nigeria. Afr Sci. 2023;24(4):504–16.

9. Andersen C, Omelekhina Y, Rasmussen BB, et al. Emissions of soot, PAHs, ultrafine particles, NOx, and other health relevant compounds from stressed burning of candles in indoor air. Indoor Air. 2021;31:2033–48. https://doi.org/10.1111/ina.12909.

10. Muhyideen O, Lukman S, Ajibola YF, Okechukwu IP. Assessment of mutagenicity and carcinogenicity risks and source apportionment of polycyclic aromatic hydrocarbons of monitored black carbon (soot) in air and swimming pool water in Port Harcourt. Res Sq, Posted 05 May, 2023. 2023; https://doi.org/10.21203/rs.3.rs-2880375/v1.

11. Wang L, Wen W, Yan J, Zhang R, Li C, Jiang H, Chen S, Pardo M, Zhu K, Jia B, Zhang W, Bai Z, Shi L, Cheng Y, Rudich Y, Morawska L, Chen J. Influence of polycyclic aromatic compounds and oxidation states of soot organics on the metabolome of human-lung cells (A549): implications for vehicle fuel selection. Environ Sci Technol. 2023;57(51):21593–604. https://eprints.qut.edu.au/245055/

12. Liu D, Li X, Liu J, Wang F, Leng Y, Li Z, Lua P, Rose NL. Probing the occurrence, sources and cancer risk assessment of polycyclic aromatic hydrocarbons in PM2.5 in a humid metropolitan city in China. Environ Sci Process Impacts. 2024; https://doi.org/10.1039/d3em00566f.

13. Pukkala E, Martinsen JI, Lynge E, et al. Occupation and cancer—follow-up of 15 million people in five Nordic countries. Acta Oncol (Stockholm, Sweden). 2009;48:646–790.

14. Tang R, Shang J, Qiu X, Gong J, Xue T, Zhu T. Origin, structural characteristics, and health effects of atmospheric soot particles: a review. Curr Pollut Rep. 2024; https://doi.org/10.1007/s40726-024-00307-9.

15. Radosavljevic V. Urinary markers/metabolites of exposure to chemical carcinogens—new possibilities in preventive oncology. Ecotoxicol Environ Saf. 2024;269:115774.

26.1 Overview

26.1.1 Exposure of the General Population

Coke oven emissions are complex mixtures, and workers are mainly exposed to polycyclic aromatic hydrocarbons (PAHs) and additionally to arsenic, cadmium, lead, nickel, vanadium, asbestos, silicon dioxide, sulfur dioxide, and sulfuric acid [1–3].

Coke production is carcinogenic to humans and causes lung cancer [2, 4, 5]. Its most representative urinary metabolite is 1-hydroxypyrene [6].

Appendix: Exposure Evaluation Questionnaire

1. Do you work in a place where you are exposed to smoke? If you work, for how long and in what jobs?..
....
    ....
    ....

2. Do you work in factories with blast furnaces, oxygen furnaces, or electric arc furnaces? If so, when and for how long?..
    ....
    ....
    ....
    ....

V. Radosavljevic, *Assessing Human Exposure to Key Chemical Carcinogens*, https://doi.org/10.1007/978-3-031-84441-6_26

3. Do you work or live near an iron and steel foundry? If you work, how long have you been working and what jobs? If you live near an iron and steel foundry, how long have you lived there and how far from the foun dry?...

....

....

....

....

References

1. IARC. Polynuclear aromatic compounds, Part 3, industrial exposures in aluminum production, coal gasification, coke production, and iron and steel founding. IARC Monogr Eval Carcinog Risk Chem Hum. 1984;34:1–219.
2. IARC. Pentachlophenol and some related compounds. IARC Monogr Eval Carcinog Risk Chem Hum. 2019;117:1–325.
3. Gao Y, Geng MZ, Wang G, Hang Y, Ji Y, Jordan RW, Jiang S-J, Yang-Guang G, An T. Environmental and dietary exposure to 24 polycyclic aromatic hydrocarbons in a typical Chinese coking plant. Environ Pollut. 2024;346:123684. https://doi.org/10.1016/j.envpol.2024.123684.
4. Vimercati L, Bisceglia L, Cavone D, Caputi A, De Maria L, Delfino MC, Corrado V, Ferri GM. Environmental monitoring of PAHs exposure, biomarkers and vital status in coke oven workers. Int J Environ Res Public Health. 2020;17:2199. https://doi.org/10.3390/ijerph17072199.
5. Zhou Y, Li Y, Fu D, Zhang Y, Xiao K, Jiang K, Luo J, Shen G, Liu W, Tao S. Pollution characteristics and health risks of polycyclic aromatic compounds (PACs) in soils of a coking plant. Toxics. 2024;12:179. https://doi.org/10.3390/toxics12030179.
6. Radosavljevic V. Urinary markers/metabolites of exposure to chemical carcinogens—new possibilities in preventive oncology. Ecotoxicol Environ Saf. 2024;269:115774.

27.1 Overview

The products of coal tar distillation consist of a complex mixture of mono- and polycyclic aromatic hydrocarbons and resin [1]. By the 1990s, coal tar became the main source of anticorrosive coatings and wood preservatives [2].

Some authors reported very high death rates from scrotal cancer among coal tar distillers, and a French study showed a significant increase in the incidence of oral cavity and pharyngeal cancer [3, 4]. Epidemiological studies are consistent that occupational exposure during tar distillation is carcinogenic to humans and causes lung cancer [2]. Its most representative urinary metabolite is 1-hydroxypyrene [5, 6].

Appendix: Exposure Evaluation Questionnaire

1. Do you work with tar? If you work, for how long and in what jobs?
   ....
   ....

2. Do you work or live near the tar or tar resin industry and for how long? ....
   ....
   ....
   ....

3. Do you work in the parking lot, in what jobs, and for how long?......................
   ....
   ....
   ....

4. Do you work or live near the bitumen industry and for how long?
   ....
   ....

V. Radosavljevic, *Assessing Human Exposure to Key Chemical Carcinogens*,
https://doi.org/10.1007/978-3-031-84441-6_27

5. Do you work as a street vendor? If so, when and for how long?.....................
....
....
....

6. Do you work in road companies, paving streets and roads, and making side-walks, in which jobs, and for how long? ....
....
....

7. Do you work or live near the tar industry, how far, and for how long? ....
....

References

1. Betts WD. Tar and pitch. In: Kirk-Othmer encyclopedia of chemical technology. 5th ed. New York: Wiley; 1997. [Online edition].
2. IARC. Chemical agents and related occupations. IARC Monogr Eval Carcinog Risks Hum. 2012;100F:1–628.
3. Moulin JJ, Mur JM, Wild P, et al. Epidemiologic study of the mortality among the employees of a coal tar distillery. Rev Epidemiol Sante Publique. 1988;36:99–107.
4. Spencer Williams E, Mahler BJ, Van Metre PC. Cancer risk from incidental ingestion exposures to PAHs associated with coal-tar-sealed pavement. Environ Sci Technol. 2013;47:1101–9. https://doi.org/10.1021/es303371t.
5. McCormick S, Snawder JE, I-Chen C, Slone J, Calafat AM, Wang Y, Meng L, Alexander-Scott M, Breitenstein M, Johnson B, Meadows J, Estill CF. Exposure assessment of polycyclic aromatic hydrocarbons in refined 1 coal tar sealant applications. Int J Hyg Environ Health. 2022;242:113971. https://www.sciencedirect.com/science/article/pii/S1438463922000542
6. Radosavljevic V. Urinary markers/metabolites of exposure to chemical carcinogens—new possibilities in preventive oncology. Ecotoxicol Environ Saf. 2024;269:115774.

Human Exposure to Polycyclic Aromatic Hydrocarbons (Emissions from Burning Coal Indoors)

28

28.1 Overview

28.1.1 Components of Coal Emissions

During the burning of coal in small and simple home stoves for cooking and heating (China and India), a significant emission of pollutants (between 10% and 30%) are the products of incomplete combustion—carbon monoxide, nitrogen dioxide, benzene, formaldehyde, benzo[a]pyrene, 1,3-butadiene, formaldehyde, polycyclic aromatic hydrocarbons (PAHs), and particles (PM [*particulae matteriae*]) vary greatly depending on the type of coal and the burning conditions [1]. Furthermore, such coal contains pollutants such as sulfur, arsenic, lead, or mercury, which are released into the air during combustion. Combustion of coal at high temperatures results in the emission of large amounts of nitrogen oxides [2], and two types of particulate matter occur: respirable particulate matter (<10 μm, called PM10) and respirable particulate matter (<2.5 μm, called PM2.5).

28.1.2 Exposure of the General Population

28.1.2.1 Exposure to Ambient Coal Smoke

An ecological study in 8073 Spanish settlements from 1994 to 2003 [3] showed effects of the nearest combustion plant that used coal as the sole fuel source on an increased risk of lung cancer overall (OR = 1.10; 95% CI = 1.02–1.18), with a higher risk in men (OR = 1.13; 95% CI = 1.05–1.22), for overall bladder cancer (OR = 1.18; 95% CI = 1.01–1.37) with a higher risk in men at 1.22 (95% CI = 1.03–1.44), and for laryngeal cancer (OR = 1.46; 95% CI = 1.21–1.77 in men). The risk calculation was adjusted for smoking and sociodemographic variables, and there were no other nearby industries that could have biased the risk estimates.

V. Radosavljevic, *Assessing Human Exposure to Key Chemical Carcinogens*,
https://doi.org/10.1007/978-3-031-84441-6_28

28.1.2.2 Indoor Exposure

A meta-analysis from four studies conducted in China showed that the use of coal for heating and cooking among people with the GSTM1 null genotype was associated with an increased risk of lung cancer (OR = 1.64; 95% CI = 1.25–2.14) [4–6]. A large multicenter hospital-based case-control study was conducted in India with 1042 hypopharynx/larynx cancers, 635 lung cancers, and 718 matched controls [7]. Regular charcoal users, compared with never charcoal users, had a relative risk for hypopharyngeal cancer of 1.92 (95% CI = 0.67–5.54), for laryngeal cancer of 2.42 (95% CI = 0.94–6.25), and for lung cancer of 3.76 (95% CI = 64–8.63) after adjustment for tobacco smoking and other factors. The risk was directly proportional to years of coal use and for hypopharyngeal cancer—the trend probability was 0.06, for laryngeal cancer the trend was 0.05, and for lung cancer it was less than 0.01.

28.1.2.3 Coal

Coal accounts for 70–75% of energy consumption in China [8–10]. About 40% of households in rural China rely on coal for heating or cooking, especially in regions with abundant and cheap coal supplies, and about 10% of urban households use coal as their primary fuel source [11]. Outside of China, the most common household use of coal is in western India (Gujarat) [12].

28.1.3 Polycyclic Aromatic Hydrocarbons

PAHs are important components of coal emissions [13, 14] and are absorbed through the respiratory tract or can be ingested in the gastrointestinal tract. Highly lipophilic PAHs released from particles deposited in the bronchial airways are absorbed into the circulation over several hours, but PAHs released from particles in the alveolar airways are absorbed within minutes [15, 16]. Small PAH molecules (2–3 rings) are absorbed faster than larger ones [15]. Absorbed PAHs are distributed to most organs and tissues and accumulate in adipose tissue [15, 17]. Some amounts are rapidly metabolized to more soluble metabolites (phenols, dihydrodiols, phenol dihydrodiols, and epoxides), which are electrophilic, bind to DNA, and produce genotoxic effects (formation of DNA adducts) [18]. PAH metabolites (the most important 1-hydroxypyrene) are eliminated as conjugates with glutathione, sulfate, or glucuronic acid [15, 17]. Benzo[a]pyrene (PAH compound) is metabolized to benzo[a]pyrene-7,8-diol-9, 10-epoxide and forms adducts in DNA (genotoxic mechanism). PAH-epoxides (from coal emissions) play an important role in the development of lung cancer [15, 18].

In summary, there is sufficient evidence for the carcinogenicity of indoor coal burning and the development of lung cancer [19]. Its main urinary metabolite is 1-hydroxypyrene [20].

Appendix: Exposure Evaluation Questionnaire

1. Did you work in coal mining and/or processing? If so, what jobs did you work and for how long? ....
....

....
....

2. Did you live near a place where coal was mined? If so, how long did you live near such a place and how far was the place where you lived from the place where the coal was mined? ....
....

....
....

....
....

3. Did you work on the purification of waste water from the coal industry? If so, what jobs did you work for and for how long? ....
....
....

4. Have you consumed food produced in the territory where coal was once extracted and/or processed (specify when)? If so, how long have you consumed it and which foods?
....
....

....
....

....
....

5. Have you worked on the removal of tailings from the coal industry? If so, what jobs did you work for and for how long? ....
....
....

....
....

6. Did you live near a place where tailings from the coal industry were disposed of? If so, how long have you lived near such a place and how far was the place where you lived from the place where the tailings from the coal industry were disposed of? ....

....
....

....
....

7. Have you consumed food produced in the territory where tailings from the coal industry (mine) were once (specify when) disposed of? If so, how long have you consumed it and which food?...

8. Do you work in the production of carbon electrodes, asbestos, or products containing asbestos? If so, in which jobs and for how long? ....

9. Do you work or live near an aluminum mine or industry and for how long? ....

10. Do you work or live near the refinery and for how long? ....

11. Do you work or live near the metal industry, chemical industry, or electrical industry and for how long? ....

12. Do you work or live near the mineral oil industry, how far, and for how long? ....

13. Do you work in the wood industry, in what jobs, and for how long? ....

References

1. IARC. Personal habits and indoor combustions. IARC Monogr Eval Carcinog Risks Hum. 2012;100E:1–598.
2. Zhang J, Smith KR, Ma Y, et al. Greenhouse gases and other airborne pollutants from household stoves in China: a database for emission factors. Atmos Environ. 2000a;34:4537–49.
3. Garcia-Perez J, Pollan M, Boldo E, et al. Mortality due to lung, laryngeal and bladder cancer in towns lying in the vicinity of combustion installations. Sci Total Environ. 2009;407:2593–602.
4. Hosgood HD 3rd, Berndt SI, Lan Q. GST genotypes and lung cancer susceptibility in Asian populations with indoor air pollution exposures: a meta-analysis. Mutat Res. 2007;636:134–43.

5. Lan Q, He X, Costa DJ, et al. Indoor coal combustion emissions, GSTM1 and GSTT1 genotypes, and lung cancer risk: a case–control study in Xuan Wei, China. Cancer Epidemiol Biomarkers Prev. 2000;9:605–8.
6. Chen HC, Cao YF, Hu WX, et al. Genetic polymorphisms of phase II metabolic enzymes and lung cancer susceptibility in a population of Central South China. Dis Markers. 2006;22:141–52.
7. Sapkota A, Gajalakshmi V, Jetly DH, et al. Indoor air pollution from solid fuels and risk of hypopharyngeal/laryngeal and lung cancers: a multicentric case–control study from India. Int J Epidemiol. 2008;37:321–8.
8. National Bureau of Statistics. China energy statistical yearbook 2005. Beijing: China Statistics Press; 2005.
9. National Bureau of Statistics. China statistical yearbook 2006. Beijing: China Statistics Press; 2006.
10. Millman A, Tang D, Perera FP. Air pollution threatens the health of children in China. Pediatrics. 2008;122:620–8.
11. National Bureau of Statistics. The major statistics of the 2nd National Survey for Agriculture. Beijing: China Statistics Press; 2008.
12. Raiyani CV, Jani JP, Desai NM, et al. Assessment of indoor exposure to polycyclic aromatic hydrocarbons for urban poor using various types of cooking fuels. Bull Environ Contam Toxicol. 1993;50:757–63.
13. IARC. Some non-heterocyclic polycyclic aromatic hydrocarbons and some related exposures. IARC Monogr Eval Carcinog Risks Hum. 2010;92:1–853.
14. Venkatraman G, Giribabu N, Mohan PS, Muttiah B, Govindarajan VK, Alagiri M, Rahman PSA, Karsani SA. Environmental impact and human health effects of polycyclic aromatic hydrocarbons and remedial strategies: a detailed review. Chemosphere. 2024;351:141227. https://doi.org/10.1016/j.chemosphere.2024.141227.
15. Gerde P, Scott BR. A model for absorption of low-volatile toxicants by the airway mucosa. Inhal Toxicol. 2001;13:903–29.
16. WHO. Selected non-heterocyclic polycyclic aromatic hydrocarbons. Geneva: International Programme on Chemical Safety, No. Environmental Health Criteria 202; 1998.
17. Xue W, Warshawsky D. Metabolic activation of polycyclic and heterocyclic aromatic hydrocarbons and DNA damage: a review. Toxicol Appl Pharmacol. 2005;206:73–93.
18. Liu D, Li X, Liu J, Wang F, Leng Y, Li Z, Peili L, Rose NL. Probing the occurrence, sources and cancer risk assessment of polycyclic aromatic hydrocarbons in PM2.5 in a humid metropolitan city in China. Environ Sci Process Impacts. 2024; https://doi.org/10.1039/d3em00566f.
19. Radosavljević V. Urinary markers of exposure to chemical carcinogens—new guidelines in preventive oncology. Belgrade: Media Center "Defense"; 2024. (in Serbian).
20. Radosavljevic V. Urinary markers/metabolites of exposure to chemical carcinogens—new possibilities in preventive oncology. Ecotoxicol Environ Saf. 2024;269:115774.

29.1 Overview

2,3,7,8-Tetrachlorodibenzo-para-dioxin (THDD) and polychlorinated dibenzofurans (PHDBFs) are not produced commercially. THDD occurs as a contaminant in chlorophenoxy herbicides and can be produced during incineration, metal processing, and pulp bleaching [1]. The amount of congener THDD depends on the combustion process and varies greatly [2].

29.1.1 Exposure of the General Population

Sources of THDD release into the environment are grouped into four main categories: incineration sources (municipal waste, hospital waste, hazardous waste, sewage sludge), combustion sources (wood-fired cement kilns, diesel vehicles, coal-fired plants, crematoria), industrial sources (pulp and paper factories, chemical production, metal industry), and other sources (biochemical processes, photolytic processes, forest fires) [3–6]. Release of PHDF and its congeners (2,3,7,8-substituted polychlorinated dibenzo-para-dioxins [PHDD] and 2,3,4,7,8-pentachlorodibenzofuran [PeHDF]) into the environment is mainly caused by combustion and incineration (emitted from cement kilns; during metal smelting and refining; chemical production of chlorophenol, vinyl chloride; pulp bleaching, coal tar incineration) [2, 7–10]. THDD is persistent in the environment and accumulates in animal fat, and most humans are exposed to THDD as a result of consumption of meat, milk, eggs, and fish [11]. Mean levels of THDD in human tissues are in the range of 2–3 ng/kg of fat. Since the mid-1980s, mean concentrations of total THDD in the general population have decreased by two to three times. Due to their lipophilic nature and resistance to biodegradation, some PHDBFs bioaccumulate in the environment, so they are distributed in all parts of the environment (air, soil, water, sediment, and biota) [12, 13]. As a result of the accumulation of PHDD in the food chain, in foods with a high fat content (dairy products, eggs, animal fats, some fish), reducing the

© The Author(s), under exclusive license to Springer Nature
Switzerland AG 2025
V. Radosavljevic, *Assessing Human Exposure to Key Chemical Carcinogens*,
https://doi.org/10.1007/978-3-031-84441-6_29

fat content of food reduces the intake of dioxins [14]. Data on THDD lipid concentrations were collected over a 30-year period (1970–2000) among the general population in the USA, Canada, Germany, and France. Mean THDD lipid levels decreased steadily, nearly ten-fold over this time period [4]. Some US-Vietnam veterans exposed to Agent Orange had 300- to 600-fold higher lipid THDD levels many years after they left Vietnam, compared to general population values [15–18]. In Vietnam, high levels of THDD were found in soil and sediment from areas contaminated with Agent Orange 3–4 decades after contamination, and elevated concentrations were measured in food and wildlife [19], as well as in Vietnamese people from contaminated areas [20–24]. Human exposure to dioxin-like compounds mainly occurs (90%) through ingestion of food containing PHB residues. The highest exposure to THDD (10–100 times higher than average levels in the 1980s) occurred in groups of industrial workers producing phenoxy herbicides and chlorophenols [4].

2,3,7,8-Tetrachlorodibenzo-para-dioxin exhibits carcinogenicity in humans for all malignancies [25]. THDD is the urinary metabolite of THDD. Methoxy-pentachlorodibenzofuran (methoxy-penta-HDF) and dimethoxy-pentachloro-biphenyl are urinary metabolites of 2,3,4,7,8-pentachlorodibenzofuran. Methoxy-pentachlorodibenzofuran (methoxy-penta-HDF) and dimethoxy-pentachloro-biphenyl are urinary metabolites of 2,3,4,7,8-pentachlorodibenzofuran [26].

Appendix: Exposure Evaluation Questionnaire

1. Do you work with municipal waste, hospital waste, hazardous waste, and sewage sludge? If so, in which jobs and for how long? ………………………………………
   ………………
   ……………………………………………………………………………………
   ………………………………

2. Do you work in the cement industry, or with cement? If so, in what jobs and for how long? ………………………………………………………………………………
   ………………………………
   ……………………………………………………………………………………
   ………………………………

3. Do you work or live near the pulp and paper industry, chemical industry (chemical production of chlorophenol, vinyl chloride; pulp bleaching, production of phenoxy herbicides), or metal industry (smelting and refining of metals)? What jobs have you been working on and for how long? How far do you live from the mentioned industries?
   ……………………………………………………………………………………
   ………………………………
   ……………………………………………………………………………………
   ………………………………

4. Do you work or live near a coal plant? What jobs have you been working on and for how long? How far do you live from the mentioned facilities? ....
....
....
....

5. Do you use diesel vehicles or are you exposed to exhaust gases from diesel vehicles? If so, for how long and in what situations? ....
....
....
....
....

6. Do you work or live near a crematorium? What jobs have you been working on and for how long? How far do you live from the mentioned facilities? ....
....
....
....

7. Do you work or live near an incinerator? What jobs have you been working on and for how long? How far and how long have you lived from the mentioned facilities?..
....
....
....

8. In the last 3 days, have you been exposed to forest or similar fires, wood burning, photolytic, or biochemical processes accompanied by the release of gases? If so, by what processes, for how long, and in what capacity?...
....
....
....
....

9. Have you consumed egg yolks, fatty dairy products, or fish in the last 3 days? If so, in what quantities, which dairy products, and which fish? Does the fish belong to the salmonids and was it caught in estuaries? ....
....
....
....
....
....

10. Have you consumed a large amount of meat in the last 3 days? If yes, in what quantities and which meat?...
....
....
....

11. Have you consumed caviar or fish roe in the last 2 days? If so, in what quantities and where do the mentioned products come from?..

12. Have you consumed shellfish or fatty food in the last 2 days? If so, in what quantities and where do the mentioned products come from?..

13. Do you consume food produced at the sites of former incinerators, landfills, or river   sediments?...

14. Do you work or live near a secondary copper smelter? What jobs have you been working on and for how long? How far and how long have you lived from the mentioned facilities? ....

15. Do you reside or live near major roads, intersections, freight routes, or bus stations? How far and how long have you lived from the mentioned facilities? ....

16. Do you work or live near a coal-fired thermal power plant? What jobs have you been working on and for how long? How far and how long have you lived from the mentioned facilities? ....

17. Do you work or live near industrial boilers? What jobs have you been working on and for how long? How far and how long have you lived from the mentioned facilities? ....

18. Do you work or live near an iron ore sintering plant? What jobs have you been working on and for how long? How far and how long do you live from the mentioned facilities? ....
....
....
....

19. Have you stayed in the territory of Vietnam or consumed food originating from the territory of Vietnam where "Agent Orange" was used during the American-Vietnam War?

If you did stay in the incriminated areas, when and how long did you stay there and in what capacity? ....
....
....
....

If you consumed food originating from the territory of Vietnam where "Agent Orange" was used during the US-Vietnam War, when did you consume it, what type of food, and how much? ....
....
....
....

20. Do you work or live near a tannery, varnish, pigment, or paint factory? What jobs have you been working on and for how long? How far away and how long have you lived near the mentioned facilities? ....
....
....
....
....
....

21. Do you work or live near a landfill, plastic factory, or electric transformer cooling fluid (polychlorinated biphenyls) factory? What jobs have you been working on and for how long? How far away and how long have you lived near the mentioned facilities? ....
....
....
....

22. Have you breathed air filled with ash in the last 3 days? If so, when and for how long? Do you know the origin of ash?...
....
....
....
....
....

23. Do you work or live near a metal recycling center? What jobs have you been working on and for how long? How far away and how long have you lived near the mentioned facilities? ....

24. In the last 2 days, have you been intensively exposed to exhaust gases from motor vehicles or exhaust gases from organic fuel heaters? If so, when and for how long? Do you know the origin of heating element fuel? ....

25. Do you work or live near the fungicide or herbicide industry? What jobs have you been working on and for how long? How far away and how long have you lived near the mentioned facilities?.. ....

26. In the last 2 days, have you consumed food or drink (wine) from the territory where fungicides and/or herbicides were intensively applied? If so, in what quantities and where do the mentioned products come from?......................... ....

27. In the last 2 days, have you been exposed to facilities where chlorine is used? If so, when and for how long? Do you know what kind of plants, processes, or products these are?.. ....

28. Have you been exposed to (worked with) the contents of electrical transformers or capacitors in the last few days? If so, when and for how long? What exactly did you do on the said devices? ....

29. Do you work or live near a steel mill, bar smelter, or electric arc furnace plant? What jobs have you been working on and for how long? How far and for how long have you lived near the mentioned facilities? ....
....
....
....
....
....

References

1. Bock MJ, Brown LE, Wenning RJ, Bell JL. Sources of 2,3,7,8-tetrachlorodibenzo-p-dioxin and other dioxins in Lower Passaic River, New Jersey, Sediments. Environ Toxicol Chem. 2021;40(5):1499–519.
2. IARC. Polychlorinated dibenzo-para-dioxins and polychlorinated dibenzofurans. IARC Monogr Eval Carcinog Risks Hum. 1997;69:1–631.
3. Kulkarni PS, Crespo JG, Afonso CAM. Dioxins sources and current remediation technologies—a review. Environ Int. 2008;34:139–53.
4. IARC. Chemical agents and related occupations. IARC Monogr Eval Carcinog Risks Hum. 2012;100F:1–628.
5. VoPham T, Bertrand KA, Fisher JA, Ward MH, Laden F, Jones RR. Emissions of dioxins and dioxin-like compounds and incidence of hepatocellular carcinoma in the United States. Environ Res. 2022;204:112386. https://doi.org/10.1016/j.envres.2021.112386.
6. WHO. https://www.who.int/news-room/fact-sheets/detail/dioxins-and-their-effects-on-human-health. Produced on 29 November 2023. Accessed on 6 Aug 2024.
7. USEPA. Exposure and human health reassessment of 2,3,7,8-tetrachlorodiobenzo-p-dioxin (TCDD) and related compounds (September 2000 draft). Part I: estimating exposure to dioxin-like compounds. Volume 2: sources of dioxin-like compounds in the United States, EPA/600/P-00/001 Bb. Washington, DC: U.S. Environmental Protection Agency/National Center for Environmental Assessment, Office of Research and Development; 2000a.
8. World Health Organization. 2019. https://www.who/ced/phe/epe/19.4.4. Accessed on 26 June 2024.
9. Lee SJ, Ha HJ, Jho EH. Assessing ecotoxicological effects of 2,3,7,8-TCDD, 1,2,3,7,8-PeCDD, and 2,3,4,7,8-PeCDF in soil using *Allivibrio fischeri*. Appl Biol Chem. 2019;62:73. https://doi.org/10.1186/s13765-019-0478-5.
10. National Center for Biotechnology Information. PubChem compound summary for CID 42128, 2,3,4,7,8-pentachlorodibenzofuran. 2024. Retrieved August 28, 2024, from https://pubchem.ncbi.nlm.nih.gov/compound/2_3_4_7_8-Pentachlorodibenzofuran
11. Haumaru Kai Aotearoa. National Chemical Contaminants Programme. Dairy products and raw milk. Dioxin, dioxin-like PCB, and non-dioxin like polychlorinated biphenyls (indicator PCBs) results (2014/15, 2015/16, 2016/17, 2017/18, 2018/19, 2019/20, 2020/21, 2021/22 and 2022/23). New Zealand Food Safety Technical Paper No: 2024/10.
12. USEPA. Exposure and human health reassessment of 2,3,7,8-tetrachlorodiobenzo-p-dioxin (TCDD) and related compounds (September 2000 draft). Part I: estimating exposure to dioxin-like compounds. Volume 3: properties, environmental levels and background exposures, EPA/600/P-00/001 Bc. Washington, DC: U.S. Environmental Protection Agency/National Center for Environmental Assessment, Office of Research and Development; 2000b.
13. ANZG. Toxicant default guideline values for aquatic ecosystem protection: dioxins in freshwater. Canberra: Australian and New Zealand Guidelines for Fresh and Marine Water Quality. CC BY 4.0. Australian and New Zealand Governments and Australian State and Territory Governments; 2023.

14. Longstreth JD, Hushon JM. Risk assessment for 2,3,7,8-tetrachlorodibenzo-p-dioxin (TCDD). In: Tucker RE, et al., editors. Human and environmental risks of chlorinated dioxins and related compounds. New York: Plenum Press; 1983.
15. Kahn PC, Gochfeld M, Nygren M, et al. Dioxins and dibenzofurans in blood and adipose tissue of Agent Orange-exposed Vietnam veterans and matched controls. JAMA. 1988;259:1661–7.
16. Schecter A, Ryan JJ, Constable JD, et al. Partitioning of 2,3,7,8-chlorinated dibenzo-p-dioxins and dibenzofurans between adipose tissue and plasma lipid of 20 Massachusetts Vietnam veterans. Chemosphere. 1990;20:951–8.
17. Schecter A, McGee H, Stanley J, Boggess K. Dioxin, dibenzofuran, and PCB including coplanar PCB levels in the blood of Vietnam veterans in the Michigan Agent Orange Study. Chemosphere. 1992;25:205–8.
18. Michalek JE, Wolfe WH, Miner JC, et al. Indices of TCDD exposure and TCDD body burden in veterans of Operation Ranch Hand. J Expo Anal Environ Epidemiol. 1995;5:209–23.
19. Olie K, Schecter A, Constable J, et al. Chlorinated dioxin and dibenzofuran levels in food and wildlife samples in the North and South of Vietnam. Chemosphere. 1989;19:493–6.
20. Schecter A, Dai LC, Päpke O, et al. Recent dioxin contamination from Agent Orange in residents of a southern Vietnam city. J Occup Environ Med. 2001;43:435–43.
21. Schecter A, Pavuk M, Constable JD, et al. A follow-up: high level of dioxin contamination in Vietnamese from Agent Orange, three decades after the end of spraying. J Occup Environ Med. 2002;44:218–20.
22. Schecter A, Quynh HT, Pavuk M, et al. Food as a source of dioxin exposure in the residents of Bien Hoa City, Vietnam. J Occup Environ Med. 2003;45:781–8.
23. Dwernychuk LW, Cau HD, Hatfield CT, et al. Dioxin reservoirs in southern Vietnam—a legacy of Agent Orange. Chemosphere. 2002;47:117–37.
24. Schecter A, Birnbaum L, Ryan JJ, Constable JD. Dioxins: an overview. Environ Res. 2006;101:419–28.
25. Radosavljević V. Urinary markers of exposure to chemical carcinogens—new guidelines in preventive oncology. Belgrade: Media Center "Defense"; 2024. (in Serbian).
26. Radosavljevic V. Urinary markers/metabolites of exposure to chemical carcinogens—new possibilities in preventive oncology. Ecotoxicol Environ Saf. 2024;269:115774.

Human Exposure to Trichlorethylene

30

30.1 Overview

Trichlorethylene has many trade names [1].

30.1.1 Occurrence in the Environment

Trichlorethylene is widely distributed in the environment due to industrial emissions. Consumer products that contain trichlorethylene are automotive products, highly processed wood, cleaning and polishing agents, chemicals in the leather industry, adhesives, paint-related products, and lubricants [1]. The presence of trichlorethylene in the environment is in the air, 97.7%; water, 0.3%; land, 0.004%; and sediments, 0.004% [2], and the average concentrations in the air are less than micrograms per cubic meter of air, except in industrially contaminated areas [3–8]. Concentrations in urban air were about three times higher than in rural areas, and mean concentrations of trichlorethylene were highest in commercial/industrial areas and lowest in forested areas [9]. A common method for disposal of trichlorethylene is incineration after mixing with combustible fuel [1].

Indoor air concentrations of trichlorethylene can increase if trichlorethylene-contaminated water is used in the household for showering, bathing, and handwashing dishes [10, 11].

30.1.1.1 Soil

Trichlorethylene is released into the soil through industrial discharges into surface waters and leaching from landfills. The molecule, like radon, evaporates from underlying soil and groundwater and enters homes, workplaces, or schools, often undetected [12].

© The Author(s), under exclusive license to Springer Nature Switzerland AG 2025
V. Radosavljevic, *Assessing Human Exposure to Key Chemical Carcinogens*,
https://doi.org/10.1007/978-3-031-84441-6_30

30.1.1.2 Water

Due to its widespread use, trichlorethylene is often found in low concentrations in groundwater, in areas near the source of contamination, ranging from several tens of parts to several hundred micrograms per liter [13–15]. People living above TCE-contaminated groundwater are exposed to TCE through vapor intrusion. Of the 36 homes, 54.3%, 47.2%, and >84% had detectable concentrations of TCE in indoor air, outdoor air, and soil gas, respectively [16]. Similar results were recorded for surface water [17, 18] and for drinking water [19, 20].

30.1.1.3 Food

Trichlorethylene often occurs in low concentrations in food, in the range of less than micrograms per kilogram, sometimes in higher concentrations if the food originates from the area of the source of contamination [21, 22].

30.1.2 Production

30.1.2.1 Volume of Production

In general, there has been a continuous decline in demand for trichlorethylene over the years due to concerns about environmental and health implications [23, 24]. The downward trend was initiated in 1995, when the Montreal Protocol on Substances that Deplete the Ozone Layer was adopted: trichlorethylene was required in all in larger quantities as a precursor in the production of alternatives to chlorofluorocarbon and as a substitute for chemicals such as 1,1,1-trichloroethane [23]. The USA was the largest consumer of trichlorethylene in 2007, followed by Western Europe, China, and Japan [25].

Over two million pounds of TCE was released into the environment from industrial sites in 2017, and due to continuous atmospheric release and the persistence of TCE in subsurface environments, it represents one of the most significant environmental contaminants of the twentieth and twenty-first centuries [26].

Trichlorethylene is best known for its use as a solvent for cleaning and degreasing metal parts, and it has numerous other uses as an anesthetic, heat transfer medium, fat and oil extraction agent, an intermediate in the production of chlorofluorocarbons, and an ingredient in many industrial products and consumer use [6]. By 1989, about 85% of trichlorethylene produced in the USA was used for metal cleaning; the remaining 15% is equally divided between exports and various applications. The pattern in Japan was similar, with 83% and 17%, respectively. In Western Europe, 95% was used for steam degreasing and 5% for other uses [27]. Similar usage patterns were reported for Canada [28] and Finland [9, 10]. The use of trichlorethylene as a solvent in Europe declined by 85% from 1984 to 2006, with a further estimated decline of 60% from 2006 to 2010 [1]. Currently, the main use of trichlorethylene is as a raw material for the production of other chemicals, such as fluorocarbons and fluoropolymers, which are being phased out under the Montreal Protocol. About 80% of the current production in the European Union is used for this purpose [1].

30.1.2.2 Metal Degreasing

The main use of trichlorethylene was in metal degreasing in all metalworking and maintenance operations to remove oil, grease, waxes, tars, and moisture prior to final surface treatments such as galvanizing, painting, anodizing, and conversion coating applications. Trichlorethylene is used in degreasing in five major industrial groups: furniture and fixtures, finished metal products, electrical and electronic equipment, transportation equipment, and various manufacturing industries. It is also used in the production of plastics, appliances, jewelry, automobiles, plumbing, textiles, paper, glass, and printing [1].

30.1.2.3 Chemical Cleaning Industry

Trichlorethylene is still used in stain removers before clothes are dry-cleaned or after clothes have been machine-cleaned [1].

30.1.2.4 Chemical Intermediates

Trichlorethylene is used in the production of polyvinyl chloride. The biggest use of trichlorethylene is currently as a raw material for chlorofluorocarbons and hydro-fluorocarbons [29].

30.1.2.5 Textile Industry

In the textile industry, the main use of trichlorethylene is for cleaning cotton and wool. It acts as a carrier solvent for liquid stains and as a solvent for waterless dyes [1, 29].

30.1.2.6 Consumer Products

Consumer products containing trichlorethylene include automotive products, wood finishing products, cleaners and polishes, chemicals in the leather industry, adhesives, paint-related products, and lubricants [1, 30].

30.1.2.7 Other Uses

Trichlorethylene was used as a reactant for the production of pesticide intermediates, in the chemical synthesis of flame retardant chemicals, as a solvent in the pharmaceutical industry, and as a carrier solvent in formulated consumer products such as fungicides and paint removers [29, 31].

30.1.3 Exposure of the General Population

Water and air become contaminated by releases of TCE from active industries or from hazardous waste sites. Concerns about the potential health effects of trichlorethylene began in the late 1970s [32] and the European Union began establishing regulations to protect workers from exposure to trichlorethylene in the 1980s. In the 1990s, they classified it as a carcinogen ("may cause cancer") and replaced it in many processes. The US National Toxicology Program (NTP) first listed trichlorethylene in 2000 [33] and about a decade later classified it as "reasonably expected to be a human carcinogen" [34]. The number of individuals with measurable concentrations of trichlorethylene is generally low and has declined in recent years. In the US National Health and Nutrition Examination Survey 1999–2000, blood samples were taken from 290 subjects and 88% of the samples were below the detection limit [35]. The mean concentration of trichlorethylene in the other 12% of subjects was 0.013 µg/l. In the 2005–2006 survey, all 3178 subjects had concentrations below the detection limit.

Trichloroethylene is rapidly and extensively absorbed following all routes of exposure and is primarily found in adipose tissue, the brain, muscle, heart, kidney, and liver [36, 37].

Trichlorethylene causes kidney cancer, liver cancer, and non-Hodgkin's lymphoma [38, 39]. Increased risks at other sites are also suspected, including cancers of the liver, prostate, bladder, and esophagus [1, 39]. Some findings suggested maternal residential exposure to solvents from industrial sources might be associated with elevated childhood cancer risks [40]. Its urinary metabolites are trichloroethanol (THE) and trichloroacetic acid (THAA) [41].

Appendix: Exposure Evaluation Questionnaire

1. Do you work in a carpet cleaning service? What jobs have you been working on and for how long? How far away and how long have you lived near the mentioned service? ....
   ....
   ....
   ....
   ....

2. Do you work in the industry of refrigerants (appliances or chemicals)? What jobs have you been working on and for how long? How far and how long have you lived near the listed industry? Do you consume food produced or water originating from the territory where the mentioned industry was or is loca ted?..
   ....
   ....
   ....
   ....

3. Do you work in the degreasing, thinner or degreasing solvent industry? What jobs have you been working on and for how long? How far and how long have you lived near the listed industry? Do you consume food produced or water originating from the territory where the mentioned industry was or is loca ted?..
   ....
   ....
   ....
   ....

4. Do you work in the chemical paint and varnish remover industry or in the adhesive industry? What jobs have you been working on and for how long? How far and how long have you lived near the listed industry? Do you consume food produced or water originating from the territory where the mentioned industry was or is located?

   ....

   ....

   ....

   ....

5. Do you work in the chemical metal tool cleaner, cleaning wipes or chemical stain remover industry? What jobs have you been working on and for how long? How far and how long have you lived near the listed industry? Do you consume food produced or water originating from the territory where the mentioned industry was or is located? ....

   ....

   ....

   ....

   ....

   ....

6. Do you work in a dry cleaning service? What jobs have you been working on and for how long? How far away and how long have you lived near the mentioned service?.....................................

   ....

   ....

   ....

   ....

7. Did you work on oiling weapons, tools, or other equipment in the army? If so, what jobs exactly did you work for and how long? How far and how long have you lived near the activity? Do you consume food produced or water originating from the territory where the mentioned activity was or is being carried out?

   ....

   ....

   ....

   ....

   ....

8. Are there people suffering from kidney, liver, prostate, esophagus, or non-Hodgkin's lymphoma in your business or residence environment? If they exist, how long have they been working with you or living in your environment? ......

   ....

   ....

   ....

   ....

9. Do you work in the production of liquid for correction of written material, industries: wood finishing, cleaning agents, polishing agents, or lubricants? What jobs have you been working on and for how long? How far and how long have you lived near the listed industries? Do you consume food produced or water originating from the territory where the mentioned industries were or are located?..

   ....

   ....

   ....

   ....

10. Do you work in the textile dyeing, printing, or laundry/cleaning industries? What jobs have you been working on and for how long? How far and how long have you lived near the listed industries? Do you consume food produced or water originating from the territory where the mentioned industries/businesses were or are located?........................

    ....

    ....

    ....

    ....

11. Do you work on cleaning/degreasing in the industry: electronics, microelectronics, telecommunications, optics, rubber and rubber products, mineral products, transport equipment, or metal products? What jobs have you been working on and for how long? How far and how long have you lived near the listed industries? Do you consume food produced or water originating from the territory where the mentioned industries/businesses were or are located?..

    ....

    ....

    ....

    ....

12. Do you work in the aviation industry, the watch industry, or the weapons industry? What jobs have you been working on and for how long? How far and how long have you lived near the listed industries? Do you consume food produced or water originating from the territory where the mentioned industries/businesses were or are located?..................................

    ....

    ....

    ....

    ....

13. Do you work in the pesticide, distillery, marine equipment, oil refining, radar, or footwear industries? What jobs have you been working on and for how long? How far and how long have you lived near the listed industries? Do you consume food produced or water originating from the territory where the mentioned industries/businesses were or are located? ....

    ....

....

....

....

....

14. Do you work in embalming, with resins, construction or maintenance of sewage, silk industry, taxidermy of birds and animals, or maintenance of work systems? What jobs have you been working on and for how long? How far and how long have you lived near the listed industries? Do you consume food produced or water originating from the territory where the mentioned industries/businesses were or are located?

....

....

....

....

15. Do you work in waste or landfill work, or as a tobacco denicotinizer? What jobs exactly have you been working on and for how long? How far and how long have you lived near the listed industries? Do you consume food produced or water originating from the territory where the mentioned industries/businesses were or are located?.......

....

....

....

....

16. Do you live in a place where there used to be a military base, military warehouses, or any of the listed incriminated industries/businesses? If you live in such a place, which of the incriminated activities were carried out there, for how long, and how much time has passed since then? ....

....

....

....

17. Are there children in your area with rhabdomyosarcomas (malignant diseases of the soft tissues of children) or children with brain tumors? If so, do they live near the incriminated industries (places) and for how long? Did their mothers live in such places during pregnancy? ....

....

....

....

....

References

1. IARC. Trichloroethylene, tetrachloroethylene and some other chlorinated agents. IARC Monogr Eval Carcinog Risks Hum. 2014;106:1–525.
2. Boutonnet JC, De Rooij C, Garny V, et al. Euro Chlor risk assessment for the marine environment OSPARCOM Region: North-sea trichloroethylene. Environ Monit Assess. 1998;53:467–87.
3. Rich AL. Air emissions from natural gas exploration and mining in the Barnett shale geologic reservoir, Unpublished dissertation. Arlington: University of Texas; 2011.
4. Wu CF, Liu LJ, Cullen A, et al. Spatial-temporal and cancer risk assessment of selected hazardous air pollutants in Seattle. Environ Int. 2011;37:11–7.
5. Billionnet C, Gay E, Kirchner S, et al. Quantitative assessments of indoor air pollution and respiratory health in a population-based sample of French dwellings. Environ Res. 2011;111:425–34.
6. Okada Y, Nakagoshi A, Tsurukawa M, et al. Environmental risk assessment and concentration trend of atmospheric volatile organic compounds in Hyogo Prefecture, Japan. Environ Sci Pollut Res Int. 2012;19:201–13.
7. Ramírez N, Cuadras A, Rovira E, et al. Chronic risk assessment of exposure to volatile organic compounds in the atmosphere near the largest Mediterranean industrial site. Environ Int. 2012;39:200–9.
8. Forand SP, Lewis-Michl EL, Gomez MI. Adverse birth outcomes and maternal exposure to trichloroethylene and tetrachloroethylene through soil vapor intrusion in New York State. Environ Health Perspect. 2012;120:616–21.
9. Wu C, Schaum J. Exposure assessment of trichloroethylene. Environ Health Perspect. 2000;108(Suppl 2):359–63.
10. Mroueh UM. Solvent use in Finland. Helsinki: National Board of Waters and the Environment; 1993.
11. Ömür-Özbek P, Gallagher DL, Dietrich AM. Determining human exposure and sensory detection of odorous compounds released during showering. Environ Sci Technol. 2011;45:468–73.
12. Ray Dorsey E, Zafara M, Lettenberger SE, Pawlik ME, Kinel D, Frissen M, Schneider RB, Kieburtz K, Tanner CM, De Miranda BR, Goldman SM, Bloem BR. Trichloroethylene: an invisible cause of Parkinson's disease? J Parkinsons Dis. 2023;13:203–18. https://doi.org/10.3233/JPD-225047.
13. Bi E, Liu Y, He J, et al. Screening of emerging volatile organic contaminants in shallow groundwater in east China. Ground Water Monit Remediat. 2012;32:53–8.
14. Fan C, Wang GS, Chen YC, Ko CH. Risk assessment of exposure to volatile organic compounds in groundwater in Taiwan. Sci Total Environ. 2009;407:2165–74.
15. Moran MJ, Zogorski JS, Squillace PJ. Chlorinated solvents in groundwater of the United States. Environ Sci Technol. 2007;41:74–81.
16. Archer NP, Bradford CM, Villanacci JF, Crain NE, Corsi RL, Chambers DM, Burk T, Blount BC. Relationship between vapor intrusion and human exposure to trichloroethylene. J Environ Sci Health A Tox Hazard Subst Environ Eng. 2015;50(13):1360–8. https://doi.org/10.1080/10934529.2015.1064275.
17. Huybrechts T, Dewulf J, Van Langenhove H. Priority volatile organic compounds in surface waters of the southern North Sea. Environ Pollut. 2005;133:255–64.
18. Burton DT, Dilorenzo JL, Shedd TR, Wrobel JG. Aquatic hazard assessment of a contaminated surficial aquifer discharge into the Bush river, Maryland (U.S.A). Water Air Soil Pollut. 2002;139:159–82.

19. Soh SC, Abdullah MP. Determination of volatile organic compounds pollution sources in Malaysian drinking water using multivariate analysis. Environ Monit Assess. 2007;124:39–50.
20. Costas K, Knorr RS, Condon SK. A case-control study of childhood leukemia in Woburn, Massachusetts: the relationship between leukemia incidence and exposure to public drinking water. Sci Total Environ. 2002;300:23–35.
21. Fleming-Jones ME, Smith RE. Volatile organic compounds in foods: a five year study. J Agric Food Chem. 2003;51:8120–7.
22. UK Health Security Agency. Guidance. Trichloroethylene: toxicological overview. Updated 10 June 2021. https://www.gov.uk/government/publications/trichloroethylene-properties-incident-management-and-toxicology/trichloroethylene-toxicological-overview. Accessed on 27 June 2024.
23. NICNAS; National Industrial Chemicals Notification and Assessment Scheme. Trichloroethylene: priority existing chemical assessment report no. 8. Sydney, Australia. 2000. Available at http://www.nicnas
24. KEMI; Swedish Chemicals Agency. Chlorinated solvents. 2012. Available at http://www.kemi.se/en/Content/Statistics/Statistics-in-brief/Statistics-in-brief%2D%2D-Substances-and-substance-groups/Chlorinated-solvents/. Accessed 19 Nov 2013.
25. Glauser J, Ishikawa Y. Chemical economics handbook marketing research report: C2 chlorinated solvents. Menlo Park: SRI Consulting; 2008. Available at http://chemical.ihs.com/nl/Public/2008Aug.pdf. Accessed 15 Nov 2013.
26. De BR, Miranda JT, Greenamyre. Trichloroethylene, a ubiquitous environmental contaminant in the risk for Parkinson's disease. Environ Sci Process Impacts. 2020;22(3):543–54. https://doi.org/10.1039/c9em00578a.
27. Mertens JA. Chlorocarbons and chlorohydrocarbons. In: Kroschwitz JI, Howe-Grant M, editors. Kirk-Othmer encyclopedia of chemical technology. 4th ed. New York: Wiley; 1993. p. 40–50.
28. Moore OR, Walker SL, Ansari R. Canadian water quality guidelines for trichloroethylene, Scientific series no. 183. Ottawa: Water Quality Branch, Inland Waters Directorate; 1991.
29. Doherty RE. A history of the production and use of carbon tetrachloride, tetrachloroethylene, trichloroethylene and 1,1,1-trichloroethane in the United States, part 2 trichloroethylene and 1,1,1-trichloroethane. J Environ Foren. 2000;1:82–93.
30. ATSDR; Agency for Toxic Substances and Disease Registry. Toxicological profile for tetrachloroethylene. Atlanta: Agency for Toxic Substances and Disease Registry, US Department of Health and Human Services, Public Health Service; 1997. p. 1–318. Available at http://www.atsdr.cdc.gov/toxprofiles/tp.as-p?id=265&tid=48. Accessed 19 Nov 2013.
31. EPA. Locating and estimating air emissions from sources of perchloroethylene and trichloroethylene. No. EPA-450/2-89-013; 1989.
32. Birkenfeld F, Gastl D, Heblich D, et al. Product ban versus risk management by setting emission and technology requirements: the effect of different regulatory schemes taking the use of trichloroethylene in Sweden and Germany as an example, Diskussionsbeitrag Nr. V-37-0. Universitat Passau; 2005.
33. NTP; National Toxicology Program. Final report on carcinogens background document for trichloroethylene. Research Triangle Park: National Toxicology Program; 2000. Available at http://ntp.niehs.nih.gov/ntp/newhomeroc/roc10/trichloro-ethylene.pdf
34. NTP; National Toxicology Program. NTP 12th report on carcinogens. Rep Carcinog. 2011;12:iii–499.
35. Jia C, Yu X, Masiak W. Blood/air distribution of volatile organic compounds (VOCs) in a nationally representative sample. Sci Total Environ. 2012;419:225–32.
36. Kroneld R. Volatile pollutants in the environment and human tissues. Bull Environ Contam Toxicol. 1989;42:873–7.

37. Coopman VAE, Cordonnier JA, De Letter EA, Piette MHA. Tissue distribution of trichloroethylene in a case of accidental acute intoxication by inhalation. Forensic Sci Int. 2003;134:115–9.

38. Dumas O, Despreaux T, Perros F, Lau E, Andujar P, Humbert M, Montani D, Descatha A. Respiratory effects of trichloroethylene. Respir Med. 2018;134:47–53. https://doi.org/10.1016/j.rmed.2017.11.021.

39. Radosavljević V. Urinary markers of exposure to chemical carcinogens—new guidelines in preventive oncology. Belgrade: Media Center "Defense"; 2024. (in Serbian).

40. Chen Y, Van Deventer D, Nianogo R, Vinceti M, Kang W, Cockburn M, Federman N, Heck JE. Maternal residential exposure to solvents from industrial sources during pregnancy and childhood cancer risk in California. Int J Hyg Environ Health. 2024;259:114388. https://doi.org/10.1016/j.ijheh.2024.114388.

41. Radosavljevic V. Urinary markers/metabolites of exposure to chemical carcinogens—new possibilities in preventive oncology. Ecotoxicol Environ Saf. 2024;269:15774.

Exposure Evaluation Questionnaires

Chapter 1

1. Do you take nutritional supplements (minerals, vitamins, elements)?   Yes   No
   How often do you take them:
   (a) Daily
   (b) Three times a week
   (c) Once a week or less often
   List what nutritional supplements you take: ....
   ....
   ....
   ....
2. How often do you stay in a smoking room for more than two hours?
   (a) Daily
   (b) Three times a week
   (c) Once a week or less often
3. Daily intake of tap water in liters: ....
   ....
4. Daily intake of other liquids in liters (bottled water, juices, beer)......................
   ....
   ....
   ....
   ....
   ....

© The Author(s), under exclusive license to Springer Nature
Switzerland AG 2025
V. Radosavljevic, *Assessing Human Exposure to Key Chemical Carcinogens*,
https://doi.org/10.1007/978-3-031-84441-6

Chapter 2

1. Do you consume sweets additionally (in addition to regular meals) and how much in grams or teaspoons (coffee with sugar, added sugar to drinks—lemonade, diluted juices, cakes, cakes)? ....

2. Do you consume sweets with rice and how much—(a) several times a day, (b) once daily, (c) three times a week, and (d) once a week—and in what quantity in grams?...............................

3. Are the sweets you consume wrapped in foil? ....Yes   No.........

4. Do you consume extra (in addition to regular meals) and how much in pieces: carrots, cucumbers, onions (summer or winter salads)? ....
...........Yes...No

5. If the previous answer is Yes, how many times do you consume—(a) several times a day, (b) once a day, (c) three times a week, and (d) once a week—and in what quantity in pieces?.................

6. Do you consume apple juice and how much—(a) several times a day, (b) once daily, (c) three times a week, and (d) once a week—and in what quantity in milliliters?...

7. Do you consume orange juice and how much—(a) several times a day, (b) once daily, (c) three times a week, and (d) once a week—and in what quantity in milliliters?............................

8. Do you consume peach juice and how much—(a) several times a day, (b) once daily, (c) three times a week, and (d) once a week—and in what quantity in milliliters?...

9. Are the juices you consume or any other type of food from Tetra Pak packaging?.................

10. How often do you eat pastries—(a) several times a day, (b) once daily, (c) three times a week, and (d) once a week—and in what quantity in grams?.................
....

11. How often do you eat bread and what kind—(a) several times a day and (b) once a day—and in what amount in grams?.................
....

12. Do you consume seafood and/or fish?   Yes   No

13. If you consume seafood and/or fish, how often:
    (a) Daily
    (b) Three times a week
    (c) Once a week or less often

14. Do you consume sauces and which ones: Yes   No ....
....

15. If you consume sauces, how often:
    (a) Daily
    (b) Three times a week
    (c) Once a week or less often

Chapter 3

1. Do you consume cereals (corn, wheat, oatmeal) and how often:
   (a) Several times every day
   (b) Once a day
   (c) Three times a week
   (d) Once a week and less often
   And in what quantity do you consume cereals? ....
   ....

2. Do you consume paprika and how often:
   (a) Daily
   (b) Three times a week
   (c) Once a week or less often

3. Do you consume chocolate and how often:
   (a) Daily
   (b) Three times a week
   (c) Once a week or less often

4. Do you consume canned fish and how often:
   (a) Daily
   (b) Three times a week
   (c) Once a week or less often

5. Do you consume sugar and how often:
   (a) Several times every day
   (b) Once a day
   (c) Three times a week
   (d) Once a week or less often
   And how much sugar do you consume? ....
   ....

6. Do you consume potatoes and how often:
   (a) Several times every day
   (b) Once a day
   (c) Three times a week
   (d) Once a week and less often
   And in what quantity do you consume potatoes? ....
   ....

7. Do you consume raspberries and how often:
   (a) Several times every day
   (b) Once a day
   (c) Three times a week
   (d) Once a week and less often
   And in what quantity do you consume raspberries? ....
   ....

8. Do you consume strawberries and how often:
   (a) Several times every day
   (b) Once a day
   (c) Three times a week
   (d) Once a week and less often
   And in what quantity do you consume strawberries? ....
   ....

9. Do you consume beets and how often:
   (a) Several times every day
   (b) Once a day
   (c) Three times a week
   (d) Once a week and less often
   And in what quantity do you consume beets?...
   ....

10. Do you consume carrots and how often:
    (a) Several times every day
    (b) Once a day
    (c) Three times a week
    (d) Once a week and less often
    And in what quantity do you consume carrots? ....
    ....

11. Do you consume tomatoes and how often:
    (a) Several times every day
    (b) Once a day
    (c) Three times a week
    (d) Once a week and less often
    And in what quantity do you consume tomatoes? ....
    ....

Chapter 4

1. Do you consume milk and dairy products (yogurt, sour milk, cheeses) and
   how often:
   (a) Several times every day
   (b) Once a day
   (c) Three times a week
   (d) Once a week and less often
   And in what quantity do you consume milk and milk products (specify which
   ones)?......................................
   ....
   ....

2. Do you consume meat and meat products (cured meat products) and how often:
   (a) Several times every day
   (b) Once a day
   (c) Three times a week
   (d) Once a week and less often
   And in what quantity do you consume meat and meat products (specify which ones)?..
   ....
   ....

3. Do you consume leafy vegetables and their products (lettuce, cabbage, kale, Swiss chard) and how often:
   (a) Several times every day
   (b) Once a day
   (c) Three times a week
   (d) Once a week and less often
   And in what quantity do you consume them (specify which leafy vegetables)?...
   ....
   ....

4. Do you consume legumes and their products (peas, green beans, beans) and how often:
   (a) Several times every day
   (b) Once a day
   (c) Three times a week
   (d) Once a week and less often
   And in what quantity do you consume them (specify which leguminous vegetables)?..
   ....
   ....

5. Do you consume other vegetables and products from other types of vegetables (fresh, canned, frozen, pasteurized) and how often:
   (a) Several times every day
   (b) Once a day
   (c) Three times a week
   (d) Once a week and less often
   And in what quantity do you consume vegetables and vegetable products (specify which ones)?..................................
   ....
   ....

6. Do you consume nuts and their products (walnuts, hazelnuts, almonds, peanuts, etc.) and how often:
   (a) Several times every day
   (b) Once a day
   (c) Three times a week
   (d) Once a week and less often
   And in what quantity do you consume nuts and products thereof (specify which ones)?......................
   ....
   ....

7. Do you consume other fruits and other fruit products (fresh, canned, frozen, pasteurized) and how often:
   (a) Several times every day
   (b) Once a day
   (c) Three times a week
   (d) Once a week and less often
   And in what quantity do you consume fruit and fruit products (specify which ones)? ....
   ....
   ....

8. Do you use oral contraceptives: Yes   No
9. If the previous answer is Yes, state which contraceptives you use and how often?
   ....
   ....

Chapter 5

1. Do you consume bananas and how often:
   (a) Several times every day
   (b) Once a day
   (c) Three times a week
   (d) Once a week or less often
   And in what quantity do you consume bananas? ....
   ....

2. Do you consume mushrooms and how often:
   (a) Several times every day
   (b) Once a day
   (c) Three times a week
   (d) Once a week or less often
   And in what quantity do you consume mushrooms? ....
   ....

3. Do you consume pears and how often:
   (a) Several times every day
   (b) Once a day
   (c) Three times a week
   (d) Once a week or less often
   And in what quantity do you consume pears?..
   ....

4. Do you consume pumpkins and how often:
   (a) Several times every day
   (b) Once a day
   (c) Three times a week
   (d) Once a week and less often
   And in what quantity do you consume pumpkins? ....
   ....

5. Do you consume tomato juice and how often:
   (a) Several times every day
   (b) Once a day
   (c) Three times a week
   (d) Once a week and less often
   And how much tomato juice do you consume? ....

6. Do you consume lemon or lemon juice (lemonade) and how often:
   (a) Several times every day
   (b) Once a day
   (c) Three times a week
   (d) Once a week or less often
   And in what quantity do you consume lemon or lemon juice (lemonade)? ....
   ....

Chapter 6

1. Have you worked in the wood protection industry or in the wood industry in general, the paint and pigment industry, metal chroming industry, leather industry, alloy industry, or paper and pulp industry?
2. If you have worked in any of the abovementioned industries, please indicate how long you have worked there and in which jobs exactly ....
   ....
   ....
   ....
   ....
   ....

3. If you lived near any of the abovementioned industries, state how long you lived there and whether you visited the mentioned industries ....
....
....
....

4. Did you consume vegetables, beans, and cereals in larger quantities than usual (when and how much)?...
....
....

5. Do you suffer from asthma or anemia (when did your illness start)?...................
....
....
....

6. In the last week, have you noticed irritation of the nose, eyes, or skin?...............................

Chapter 7

1. In the last few days, have you had nausea, unsteady gait, loss of appetite, lethargy, jaundice, stomach pain, swelling, or spontaneous bleeding? ....
....
....
....

2. Have you consumed nuts (Brazilian, Indian, European) in the last few days and how often:
   (a) Daily
   (b) Three times a week
   (c) Once a week or less often

3. Have you consumed seeds (rich in oil) in the last few days and how often:
   (a) Daily
   (b) Three times a week
   (c) Once a week or less often

4. If you consume corn and corn products, how often:
   (a) Daily
   (b) Three times a week
   (c) Once a week or less often

5. If you consume peanuts, pistachios, and/or hazelnuts, how often:
   (a) Daily
   (b) Three times a week
   (c) Once a week or less often

6. If you consume apricots, figs, mulberries, dates, and/or sugar from Chinese cane, how often:
   (a) Daily
   (b) Three times a week
   (c) Once a week or less often

7. If you consume rice and/or rice foods, how often:
   (a) Daily
   (b) Three times a week
   (c) Once a week or less often
8. If you consume pastries, how often:
   (a) Daily
   (b) Three times a week
   (c) Once a week or less often
9. If you consume soy and/or soy products, how often:
   (a) Daily
   (b) Three times a week
   (c) Once a week or less often
10. If you consume milk, yogurt, cheese, baby milk, powdered milk, flavored milk, and/or other dairy products, how often:
    (a) Daily
    (b) Three times a week
    (c) Once a week or less often
11. Do you consume any other cereals and how often:
    (a) Daily
    (b) Three times a week
    (c) Once a week or less often

Chapter 8

1. During the last few days, have you smoked or been exposed to tobacco smoke and to what extent? ....

2. During the last few days, were you exposed to oil fumes during frying for several hours and to what extent? ....

3. During the last few days, have you been exposed to aniline dyes or dyes in general and to what extent? ....

4. During the last few days, have you been exposed to hair dyes and to what extent? ....

5. During the last few days, have you sprayed apples or other fruits against fungi and to what extent? ....

6. Do you consume food containing colors and how often: ....
....
....
....
   (a) Daily
   (b) Three times a week
   (c) Once a week or less often
7. Do you use cosmetic products that contain colors and how often: ....
....
....
....
   (a) Daily
   (b) Three times a week
   (c) Once a week or less often
8. Do you use colored laundry and how often: ....
....
....
....
   (a) Daily
   (b) Three times a week
   (c) Once a week or less often

Chapter 9

1. Have you used slimming products?   (a) Yes   (b) No
2. If you used slimming products, which ones and for how long? ....
....
....
3. In the last week, have you consumed bulb vegetables, cucumber, or lettuce every
   day (which ones and for how long)?..
....
....
4. Do you suffer from chronic kidney failure and/or urinary tract cancer? ....
....
5. Are there people in your area suffering from chronic kidney failure and/or urinary tract cancer and in what number? ....
....
....
6. Do you live in an area known for suffering from Balkan endemic nephropathy
   (how long)?...
....

Chapter 10

1. During the last week, were you exposed to fire and for how long?......................
....

2. Are you employed and in what jobs in:
   - Oil, natural gas, or refineries industry
   - Chemical industry (specify what type of chemical industry, pay particular attention to the styrene or Styrofoam industry) ....
   ....
   - Footwear industry
   - Rubber industry
   - Printers

3. During the last week, have you been exposed to:
   - Colors
   - Varnishes
   - Nail polish remover
   - Industrial solvents
   - Gasoline and other fuels
   - Glues
   - Furniture wax
   - Detergents
   - Adhesives and coatings
   - Tires
   - Crude oil
   - Means for industrial cleaning and degreasing
   - Exhaust gases of motor vehicles (at least 1 h a day)

4. During the last week, have you been near landfills and/or gas stations and for how long? ....
....
....

5. Are you a smoker or have you been exposed to tobacco smoke in the last few days?..............
....
....

6. Have you consumed smoked or canned fish in the last few days and in what quantity? ....

7. Have you consumed greasy salads (Russian, French, chicken, tzatziki, etc.) in recent days and in what quantity? ....
....
....
....

8. Have you consumed smoked, cured meat, fermented, and/or preserved meat in the last days and in what quantity? ....
....
....
....

9. Have you consumed the following spices, vanilla, mint, orange concentrate, hazelnuts, chocolate, pistachios, cola, and concentrated fruit juices, in the last few days? Which and in which faces?..
....
....
....

10. Have you consumed food in the last few days to which benzoates, benzoic acid, vitamin C, and acidity regulators have been added, and in what quantity? ....
....
....

Chapter 11

1. Have you been in contact with colors, in particular azo dyes? When, how, and how long? ....
....

2. Have you been in contact with colored leather or textiles, esp. azo dyes? When, in what way, and for how long? ....
....
....

3. Have you been in contact with paper dyes or colored paper (esp azo dyes)? When, in what way, and for how long? ....

4. Have you been in contact with colored toys, esp. azo dyes? When, in what way, and for how long? ....

5. Did you live near paint factories, especially azo dye? When, in what way, and for how long? ....

Chapter 12

1. Are you exposed to burning wood or coal? When, how often, and in what situation-pit? ....
....

2. Are you exposed to machine oil? When, how often, and in what situations?..........
....
....

3. Do you work or live near thermal power plants or coal mines?

4. Do you work or live near a factory and what kind? ....

5. Do you work or live near a landfill and what kind? ....

6. Are you exposed to exhaust gases from motor vehicles? In what way and how much time a day?..
....

7. Are you exposed to biomass burning? In what way and how much time a day?.
....
....

8. Do you work or live near a metal industry and what kind?...................................
....
....

9. Do you work or live in a rural or urban environment? ....
....
....

10. Do you live or work in blocks of buildings along boulevards or important roads?
....
....
....
....

11. Do you live or work near large parking lots or intersections?
....
....

12. Do you live or work near railway (tram) stations or near traffic tracks? ....
....
....
....

13. Do you have a garden next to roads (roads or railways) or streets?.............
....
....

14. Are there people in your neighborhood or colleagues at work suffering from
lung, skin, or bladder cancer? ....
....

15. Have there been any cases of premature or mentally handicapped children in
your neighborhood? ....
....

16. Do you use water from rivers and/or lakes that are in the immediate vicinity of
landfills, metal industries, thermal power plants, coal mines, refineries, or
chemical industries?
....
....

17. In the last week, have you consumed oils, fats, smoked fish and/or meat, sweets,
or other highly processed cereal products? If so, specify which ones, when, and
how much?

18. Were you exposed to tobacco smoke during the previous 5 days and to
what extent?
....
....

19. Do you work in the construction of roads and sidewalks (especially during the last 10 days)?
....
....

20. Do you work as a truck, bus driver or have you had long drives in motor vehicles in the last week? ....
....
....

21. Are you a traffic driver or a chimney sweep, or do you work in the coal industry or in wood impregnation? ....
....

22. Did you consume grilled meat, spring barley during the last week, or drinks made from wild barley (when and in what quantity)?...
....
....

Chapter 13

1. Do you work in a chemical laboratory and in what jobs?...............................
....
....

2. Do you work in the textile industry and in what jobs?...................................
....
....

3. Do you work in the pulp and/or Styrofoam industry and in what jobs?.................
....
....

4. Do you work in the rubber industry and in what jobs?...................................
....
....
....

5. Do you work in the resin and polymer industry and in what jobs?.....................
....
....
....

6. Do you work in the industry of plastics and/or waterproof materials and in which position?
Hunting? ....
....
....
....

7. Do you work in the chlorine industry and in what jobs?.......................................
....
....
....

Chapter 14

1. Are you a tobacco user? ....
2. Do you work or live near an oil refinery? ....
3. Do you work or live near the synthetic materials industry, especially synthetic rubber and thermoplastic resins? ....
....
....
4. Do you work or live near a landfill for synthetic materials? ....
....
....
5. Do you work or live near major roads? ....
....
6. Are you exposed to exhaust gases from motor vehicles and for how long?
....
....
7. Do you work in the oil and gas extraction industry or do you live near an oil and gas extraction facility? ....
....
....
....
8. Are you exposed to stubble burning or other burnings in agriculture and how much?..
....
9. Are you exposed to forest fires or the burning of bushes or other vegetation and how much?..
....
10. Do you work or live near a landfill? ....
11. Were you exposed to burning biomass (wood, leaves, twigs, straw), when, and for how long? ....
....
12. Do you work or live near a plant where oil is heated at high temperatures? ......
....
13. Do you work or live near a plant where paper or cardboard is produced? ....
....

14. Are you often exposed to electrosurgical procedures and how much?................
....

....

....
15. Do you work or live near a coal mine?...
16. Do you work as a hairdresser? ....

Chapter 15

1. Do you work or live near plastic factories or landfills? ....
....

2. Do you work or live near the oil shale industry? ....
....

3. Do you work or live near plastic resin factories? ....
....

4. Do you work or live near factories that use plastic in any way? ....
....

....
5. Are you in any intensive contact with plastic products (food packaging, toys, household appliances, etc.)? ....
....

....

....

Chapter 16

1. Are you in any contact with industrial waxes or preparations containing them? Specify which preparations, type, and time of contact ....
....

....

....
2. Are you in any contact with chemical sealants or preparations containing them? Specify which preparations, type, and time of contact ....
....

....

....
3. Do you work or live near chlorinated solvents, plastics, lubricants and oils, or rubber industries? Specify the type of industry, type, and time of exposure..
....

....

....

....

4. Are you in any contact with stain removers, paraffin removers, cleaning or degreasing agents, galvanizers, or preparations containing them? Specify which preparations, type, and time of contact ....
....
....
....

5. Do you work or live near a place where waste is incinerated? Specify the type of incinerator, type, and time of exposure ....
....
....
....

6. Do you work or live near a place where there is intensive burning of motor fuels? Specify the type, and time of exposure ....
....
....
....

7. Do you work or live near the place where there is a gas station? Specify the type and time of exposure ....
....
....
....

8. Have you been exposed to fumigants? Specify the type and time of exposure ....
....
....
....

9. Have you been exposed to paint removers, varnishes, or means for removing the finish of furniture? Specify the type and time of exposure ....
....
....
....

10. Have you been exposed to the industry of chemical and related products, machines (except electrical), finished metal products, textile products, or photographic film? Specify the type and time of exposure ....
....
....
....

11. Do you work or live near a wastewater treatment plant? Specify the type and time of exposure ....
....
....
....

12. Is there a person in your area (family members, neighbors, colleagues at work) with detected 1,2-dichloropropane in their blood or urine? ....
....

Chapter 17

1. Did you work or live near chemical plants that produced of glycol ethers, polyglycol ethers, ethanolamines, ethoxylates, acrylonitrile, detergents, solvents, emulsifiers, fumigants, disinfection of food products? Specify the method, period (length of duration), and time (how long before sampling) of exposure ...
   ....
   ....
   ....
   ....
   ....
   ....

2. Have you been exposed **<u>tobacco smoke</u>** and/or car exhaust fumes? Specify the method, period (length of duration), and time (how long before sampling) of exposure ....
   ....
   ....
   ....
   ....

3. Have you participated in gas disinfection of medical material and/or medical equipment? Specify the method, period (length of duration), and time (how long before sampling) of exposure ....
   ....
   ....
   ....

4. Do your close relatives (parents, brothers, sisters, children) have an increased level of ethylene oxide in their urine? ....
   ....

5. Have you been exposed to the smells of ripening fruits, vegetables, or grains? Specify the method, period (length of duration), and time (how long before sampling) of exposure ....
   ....
   ....
   ....

6. Have you been exposed to the burning of fossil fuels (coal, oil, and their derivatives), pentane, or wood? Specify the method, period (length of duration), and time (how long before sampling) of exposure ....
   ....
   ....
   ....
   ....
   ....

7. Have you been exposed to fires or frying in soybean oil? Specify the method, period (length of duration), and time (how long before sampling) of exposure ....
....
....
....

8. Have you been exposed to antifreeze, glues, or working with plastic? Specify the method, period (length of duration), and time (how long before sampling) of exposure.................
....
....
....
....

Chapter 18

1. Did you work in a pesticide factory or live near a pesticide factory? If so, which pesticides, for how long, and in which jobs?..
....
....

2. Have you used pesticides in plant protection or in agriculture? If so, which pesticides did you use, for how long, and for what purposes? ....
....
....

3. Have you worked in a pesticide dump or lived near a pesticide dump? If so, which pesticides, for how long, and in which jobs?..
....
....
....

4. Did you work in a pesticide warehouse or live near a pesticide warehouse? Yes? If so, which pesticides, for how long, and in which jobs?..........................
....
....
....

5. Have you worked on disinfection jobs? If so, which pesticides did you use, for how long, and in what specific jobs did you work?..
....
....
....

6. Have you worked in pesticide destruction jobs or lived near places where pesticide destruction was carried out? If so, which pesticides, for how long, and in which jobs?..
....
....
....

7. Did you consume grains (especially rice and corn) in large quantities during the week before giving your urine for analysis? If so, which cereals, for how long, and from which areas? ....
....
....

8. Did you consume a lot of fruit during the week before giving your urine for analysis? If so, which fruit, for how long, and from which areas?......................
....
....
....

9. Did you consume a lot of vegetables during the week before giving your urine for analysis? If yes, which fruit, for how long, and from which areas?...............
....
....
....

10. Did you consume milk and/or milk products in large quantities during the week before providing your urine for analysis? If so, which products, for how long, and from which areas?..
....
....
....

11. Did you consume fish or seafood in large quantities during the week before providing your urine for analysis? If so, what kind of fish do they produce, for how long, and from which areas (rivers, seas, etc.)?...
....
....
....

12. Did you work in the wood industry or live near a wood industry factory? If so, which pesticides did you use, for how long, and in what jobs did you work?.....
....
....
....
....

13. Have you worked in, or lived near, the recycling or wastewater treatment industry? If so, were pesticides or wood recycled (were pesticides also treated and which ones)? How long and in what jobs did you work?...
....
....
....

14. Did you grow and/or sell ornamental plants? If so, which pesticides did you use, for how long, and in what jobs did you work?...
....
....

15. Have you worked on the destruction of animal ectoparasites or lived near a livestock farm where the destruction of livestock ectoparasites was carried out? If so, which pesticides did you use, for how long, and in what jobs did you work? ....

....

....

16. Have you used insecticides in the treatment of lice and scabies in humans? If so, which insecticides did you use, for how long, and in what jobs did you work?

....

....

17. Did you grow fodder plants or cultivate pastures? If so, what pesticides did you use, for how long, and what kind of work did you do?

....

....

18. Did you work in the plastics industry or live near such places, and were insecticides used there and which ones? If so, which pesticides, how long, and in what jobs did you work?...

....

....

....

19. Have you used insecticides for military purposes? If so, which insecticides, how long were they used, and what jobs did you work in?...............................

....

....

....

20. Have you been exposed to high temperatures for several hours on surfaces where pesticides were once intensively used (two or three decades ago)? If so, how long were you exposed to and to how high temperatures? What pesticides were used and for how long on such land? ....

....

....

....

21. Did you consume a lot of water during the week before giving your urine for analysis? If so, is that water from arterial wells on agricultural land? How long and in what quantity did you consume it? ....

....

22. Did you consume animal fat in a larger amount during the week before giving your urine for analysis? If so, how long and in what quantity did you consume them?

....

....

....

23. Were there floods in your area? If so, when and where did the tidal wave come from? ....
....

24. Are there any lymphoma patients in your area?...
....

25. Do you live in an urban, semi-urban, or rural settlement? ....
....

26. Do you use insecticides in your household? Which, when, in which places, and under what conditions? ....
....
....

27. Is there an intensive use of insecticides/pesticides in the area where you lived or live? If there is, when is it applied, for how long, and for what purposes? ....
....

28. Do you often consume wine and/or fruit juices? If you consume them, how often and in what quantity? ....
....
....
....

Chapter 19

1. Did you work in the polyurethane industry or live near such places, or places where polyurethane products were disposed/stored? If so, how long did you work/ live in such places and what jobs did you work in the polyurethane industry? ....
....
....

2. Did you work in the industry of urethane rubber, industrial rubber, conveyor belts, or absorbent materials (pads) or lived near such places, or places where raw materials or finished products of the mentioned industries were stored? If so, how long have you worked/lived in such places and what jobs have you held in the mentioned industries? ....
....
....
....
....
....

3. Have you worked in the waste water industry or lived near such places? If so, how long have you worked/lived in such places and what jobs have you held in the waste water industry? ....
....
....

4. Have you worked in the industry of sealants (for wood or roof structures), urethane resins, urethane resins, chipboard, insulating materials for the electrical industry, ball seals, turbines and jet engines, weapon mounts, or positioning tapes? If so, how long have you worked/lived in such places and what jobs have you held in the mentioned industries? ....
....
....
....
....
....

5. Have you worked in landfills or lived near such places? If so, how long did you work/live in such places and what jobs did you do?..
....
....
....
....
....

6. During the last week before giving the sample for analysis, did you consume turnips, cabbage, beans, turnips, cane sugar, or cucumber? If so, how often and in what quantity? ....
....
....
....
....
....

7. Have you worked in the ski equipment industry (rubber ski boots) or lived near such places? If so, how long have you worked/lived in such places and what jobs did you do?...
....
....

8. Did you work in shipyards? If so, how long have you worked in such places (watering and shaping masses/spaces) and what jobs did you do?
....
....
....
....

9. Have you worked in laboratories where 4,4′-methylenebis(2-chloroaniline) was used? If so, how long have you worked in such places and what jobs did you do?..
....
....

10. Did you work in the production of gears, polyurethane moldings or lived near such places? If so, how long have you worked/lived in such places and what jobs did you do? ....
....

11. Have you worked in the production of shoe soles, rollers and belt drives in cameras, or wheels and pulleys for escalators and elevators? If so, how long have you worked/lived in such places and what jobs did you do?............................
....
....

Chapter 20

1. Are you a smoker or are you exposed to tobacco smoke? If so, when and how much did you smoke or were you exposed to tobacco smoke? ....
....
....
....

2. Do you wear skin-tight clothing dyed with synthetic dyes? If you wear it, state when you wear it and for how long?..
....
....
....

3. If you wear clothes that stick to your skin, dyed with synthetic dyes, do you know from which country such clothes come from or who is the manufacturer?
....
....
....

4. Do you work or live near paint, rubber, motor lubricants and oil, or brake oil factories? If so, how long did you work/live in such places and what jobs did you do? ....
....
....
....
....

5. Do you use electronic cigarettes or are you exposed to their smoke? If so, when and how much did you smoke electronic cigarettes or were you exposed to their smoke? ....
....
....

6. Do you work or live near cardboard or cardboard packaging factories? If so, how long did you work/live in such places and what jobs did you do?
....
....
....
....

7. Do you often use food from cardboard packaging? If so, state when you consumed it and for how long? ....
   ....
   ....
   ....

Chapter 21

1. Do you work or live near rubber or paint and varnish factories? If so, how long did you work/live in such places and what jobs did you do?
   ....
   ....
   ....
   ....

2. Do you work in the production of ortho-toluidine? If you work, how long have you worked and what jobs have you held? ....
   ....
   ....
   ....

3. Do you work or live near organic dye or pigment factories? If so, how long did you work/live in such places and what jobs did you do?
   ....
   ....
   ....
   ....

4. Do you work or live near artificial resin or herbicide factories? If so, how long did you work/live in such places and what jobs did you do?
   ....
   ....
   ....
   ....

5. Do you work or live near indigodye or photographic dye factories? If so, how long did you work/live in such places and what jobs did you do?
   ....
   ....
   ....
   ....

6. Are you a smoker or do you stay in rooms where there is tobacco smoke? If so, how long have you worked/lived in such places? ....
   ....
   ....
   ....
   ....

7. Do you stay in rooms where there was a lot of tobacco smoke before? If so, how long have you worked/lived in such places? ....

....

....

8. Do you work or live near a wastewater treatment plant? If so, how long did you work/live in such places and what jobs did you do?

....

....

....

....

9. Do you work or stay in premises where tissue staining for microscopic preparations is performed? If so, how long have you worked in such places? ....

....

....

....

....

10. Do you work or stay in premises where blood or urine glucose analyzes are performed? If so, how long have you worked in such places? ....

....

....

11. Do you work or stay in premises where dental anesthetics (prilocaine) are applied? If so, how long have you worked in such places? ....

....

....

....

12. Do you have tattoos and when did you get them? Have you tattooed other people? If so, how long have you worked in such places?

....

....

....

....

13. Do you work or stay in premises where hair dyes or varnishes are used? If so, how long did you work/stay in such places? ....

....

....

....

....

14. Do you work or stay in premises where hair dyes are used? If so, how long did you work/stay in such places? ....

....

....

Chapter 22

1. During the last month, have you used (or been exposed to) bactericides, fungicides, herbicides, algicides, defoliants, or tree protection agents? If so, when was it and to what extent? ....
....
....
....
....

2. Do you work in the wood industry (carpentry) or in the industry of wood protection chemicals? Do you live near a wood industry or near a wood protection chemical industry? If so, when was it, how long was it, and to what extent were you exposed to the chemicals? ....
....
....
....
....
....

3. During the last week, have you consumed a large amount of pork, chicken, or river fish? If so, when was it, how many times did you consume it, and in what quantity? ....
....
....
....
....
....

4. During the last week, have you consumed a large amount of beef, mutton, offal, eggs, or poultry? If so, when was it, how many times did you consume it, and in what quantity? ....
....
....
....
....
....

5. Did you work in a fish farm? If so, when, in what jobs, and for how long?..........
....
....

6. Did you work in the furniture industry? If so, when, in what jobs, and for how long? ....
....
....
....

7. During the last week, have you consumed a large amount of seafood (shellfish, crabs, shrimps)? If so, when was it, how many times did you consume it, and in what quantity? ....
....
....
....

8. Have you worked in the industry: leather, paper, or shipyards? If so, when, in what jobs, and for how long?...
....
....
....

9. Have there been people in your environment (family members, neighbors, colleagues at work, etc.) suffering from non-Hodgkin's lymphoma? If so, who got sick and when? ....
....
....

10. Is your diet rich in animal fats? Have you consumed a large amount of animal fat during the last week? If so, when and how much?
....
....
....
....

11. Have you worked in rice fields or in swampy conditions? If so, when, in what jobs, and for how long?...
....
....
....

12. Did you work in metal mines? If so, in which mines, when, on which jobs, and for how long?...
....
....
....

13. During the last week, did you consume a large amount of river fish or fish from a pond? If so, when was it, how many times did you consume it, and in what quantity? ....
....
....
....

14. Have you worked or lived near a wastewater treatment plant? If so, in which plants, when, in which jobs, and for how long?.......................................
....
....

15. During the last week, have you consumed a large quantity of onions, lettuce, or other bulbous vegetables? If so, when was it, how many times did you consume it, and in what quantity? ....
....
....
....

16. During the last week, did you consume a large amount of milk and milk products? If so, when was it, how many times did you consume it, and in what quantity? ....
....
....
....

Chapter 23

1. During the last week, have you consumed a large amount of river fish (catfish, pike, perch) or fish from a pond? If so, when was it, how many times did you consume it, and in what quantity? ....
....
....
....
....

2. During the last week, have you consumed large amounts of sea fish (salmon, tuna, herring, mackerel, anchovies, cod, etc.) or seafood (shellfish, squid, crabs)? If so, when was it, how many times did you consume it, and in what quantity?..................................
....
....
....
....
....

3. Have you worked in the paint industry? If so, in which industries, when, in which jobs, and for how long?...
....
....
....

4. Did you live near paint factories? If so, to which paint factories, when, at what distance, and for how long?...
....
....
....

5. During the last week, have you consumed a large amount of beef steak, fried chicken, beef, eggs, or French fries? If so, when was it, how many times did you consume it, and in what quantity? ....
....
....
....
....
....

6. Have you worked in the color pigment or polymer resin industry? If so, in which industries, when, in which jobs, and for how long?.....................................
....
....
....

7. Have you lived near factories of colored pigments or polymer resins? If so, to which paint factories, when, at what distance, and for how long?.......................
....
....
....
....
....

8. During the last week, did you consume a large amount of milk and milk products? If so, when was it, which dairy products did you consume, how many times, and in what quantity? ....
....
....
....
....

9. Have you worked in the industry of plasticizers, building sealants, fluorescent lamps, or flame retardants? If so, in which industries, when, on what jobs, and for how long?..
....
....

10. Have you lived near factories for plasticizers, building sealants, fluorescent bulbs, or flame retardants? If so, in which paint factories, when, at what distance, and for how long?...
....
....
....
....

11. Did you work in the industry of transformers or capacitors, that is, in the production of liquids used for their cooling? If so, in which industries, when, in which jobs, and for how long?...
....
....
....

12. Did you live in the vicinity of transformer, condenser, or liquid production plants used for their cooling? If so, near which factories, when, at what distance, and for how long?..
....
....
....
....

13. Have you worked in the industry of adhesives, printer ink, insulators, paints, or pesticides? If so, in which industries, when, in which jobs, and for how long?
....
....
....
....

14. Have you lived near glue, printer ink, insulator, paint, or pesticide factories? If so, near which factories, when, at what distance, and for how long?..................
....
....
....
....
....

15. Have you worked in the recycling industry or in landfills? If so, in which industries, when, in which jobs, and for how long? ....
....
....
....
....
....

16. Have you lived near a recycling industry or a landfill? If so, near which factories or landfills, when, at what distance, and for how long?
....
....
....
....

17. Did you work in steel mills or were you exposed to burning coal or wood? If so, in which industries, when, in which jobs, and for how long? ....
....
....
....
....

18. Have you lived near a steel mill or a place with intensive burning of coal or wood? If so, near which steel mills or places with intensive burning of coal or wood, when, at what distance, and for how long? ....
....
....
....
....

19. Did you work in the ceramics industry or were you a ceramist? If so, in which industries, when, in which jobs, and for how long did you work?.....................
....
....
....
....
....

20. Have you worked in the electronics industry, electronic recycling centers, or the paper industry? If so, in which industries, when, in which jobs, and how long have you been working? ....
....
....
....
....

21. Have you lived near an electronic industry, electronic recycling centers, or a paper industry? If so, near which industries, when, at what distance, and for how long? ....
....
....
....
....

22. Have you lived in buildings built between 1950 and 1970? If so, when and how long did you live in them? ....
....
....
....
....

23. Have you lived or worked in dusty conditions? If so, where, when, and how long did you live there? ....
....
....
....
....

24. Have you worked in the silicone rubber or oil industry? If so, in which industries, when, in which jobs, and for how long did you work? ....
....
....
....
....
....

25. Do you live in a rural, urban, or industrial region? If in an urban or industrial region, near which industries, when, at what distance, and how long did you live there? ....
....
....

....

....

26. Are there any patients with non-Hodgkin's lymphoma in your area (neighborhood or at work)? If there are, how many are there and how much time do you spend with them or in their surroundings? ....

....

....

....

....

....

27. During the last week before the urinalysis, did you often consume fatty foods? Which one, in what quantity, and how often do you consume it? ....

....

....

....

....

....

28. Do you work in a rural, urban, or industrial region? If so, in an urban or industrial region, near which industries, when, at what distance, and how long did you work there? ....

....

....

....

....

29. Do you work with plaster or plaster? If so, in which industries, when, in which jobs, and for how long did you work? ....

....

....

....

....

....

30. Do you work in stores or in the production of TV/radio/stereo/video players/phones/tablets? If so, in which industries, when, in which jobs, and for how long did you work? ....

....

....

....

....

....

31. Do you work in the vehicle recycling industry? If so, in which industries, when, in which jobs, and for how long did you work?..

....

....

....

....

Chapter 24

1. Have you worked in the extraction and/or processing of oil shale? If so, what jobs did you work and for how long? ....

2. Did you live near a place where oil shale was extracted? If so, how long did you live near such a place and how far was the place where you lived from the place where the oil shale was extracted? ....

3. Have you worked on wastewater treatment from the oil shale industry? If so, what jobs did you work for and for how long? ....

4. Have you consumed food produced in the territory where oil (oil) shale was once extracted and/or processed (specify when)? If so, how long have you consumed it and which food? ....

5. Have you worked on the removal of waste rock (material) from the oil shale industry? If so, what jobs did you work for and for how long? ....

6. Did you live near a place where waste material from the oil shale industry was disposed of? If so, how long have you lived near such a place and how far was the place where you lived from where the waste material from the oil shale industry was disposed of? ....

7. Have you consumed food produced in the territory where tailings from the oil shale industry were once (specify when) disposed of? If so, how long have you consumed it and which food?.. ....

....

....

....

....

8. Did you work on oil extraction and/or processing? If so, what jobs did you work and for how long? ....

....

....

....

9. Did you live near a place where oil was extracted? If so, how long did you live near such a place and how far was the place where you lived from the place where the oil was extracted? ....

....

....

....

....

....

10. Have you worked on the purification of waste water from the oil industry? If so, what jobs did you work for and for how long? ....

....

....

11. Have you consumed food produced in the territory where oil extraction and/or processing was once (specify when) carried out? If so, how long have you consumed it and which food?..

....

....

....

....

....

12. Have you worked on the removal of waste materials from the oil industry? If so, what jobs did you work for and for how long? ....

....

....

....

....

13. Have you lived near a place where waste material from the oil industry was disposed of? If so, how long have you lived near such a place and how far was the place where you lived from the place where waste material from the oil industry was disposed of? ....

....

....

....

....

....

14. Have you consumed food produced in the territory where once (specify when) waste material from the oil industry was dumped? If so, how long have you consumed it and which food?...
....
....
....
....
....

15. Did you work on extracting and/or processing natural gas? If so, what jobs did you work and for how long? ....
....
....
....

16. Did you live near a place where natural gas was extracted and/or processed? If so, how long have you lived near such a place and how far was the place where you lived from where natural gas was extracted and/or processed? ....
....
....
....
....
....

17. Have you worked on wastewater treatment from the natural gas industry? If so, what jobs did you work for and for how long? ....
....
....

18. Have you consumed food produced in the territory where extraction and/or processing of natural gas was once (specify when) performed? If so, how long have you consumed it and which food?...
....
....
....
....
....

19. Have you worked on the removal of waste materials from the natural gas industry? If so, what jobs did you work for and for how long? ....
....
....
....
....

20. Have you lived near a site where waste material from the natural gas industry was disposed of? If so, how long have you lived near such a place and how far was the place where you lived from the place where waste material from the natural gas industry was disposed of?...
....

....

....

....

....

21. Have you consumed food produced in the territory where waste material from the natural gas industry was once (specify when) disposed of? If so, how long have you consumed it and which food?...

....

....

....

....

....

22. Have you used water whose source is located or transported through oil shale deposits or oil shale processing industry, coal deposits or coal processing industry, oil deposits or oil processing industry, natural gas deposits, or industry natural gas processing? If so, when and for how long?...

....

....

....

Chapter 25

1. Do you work or live in an environment with a significant presence of soot? If so, how much time do you spend daily in such an environment and how long have you lived like that?..

....

....

2. Do you work or live in a dusty environment? If so, how much time do you spend daily in such an environment and how long have you lived like that? ....

....

....

....

3. Do you work in the industry of sintering (consolidation by heating) of ores and metals? If so, in what jobs and for how long? ....

....

....

....

4. Is there a significant number of individual fireplaces in your neighborhood and what materials are used to heat them?...

....

....

....

5. Are you exposed to burning candles? If so, when and for how long?

    ....
    ....

6. Do you work in construction? If so, in what jobs and for how long?.................
    ....

    ....
    ....

7. Are you exposed to soot in any way (inhalation, ingestion, through the skin) and
    for how long? ....
    ....

    ....
    ....

    ....
    ....

8. Have you been near an open fire (burning stubble in a field, forest fires)? If so,
    when and for how long?...
    ....

    ....
    ....

9. Do you work or live near a waste incinerator and for how long? ....
    ....
    ....

    ....
    ....

10. Do you work or live near a mine or quarry and for how long? ....
    ....
    ....

11. Do you work or live near major (frequent) roads and for how long? ....
    ....
    ....

    ....
    ....

12. Do you work or live near large factory chimneys? If so, how far and for how
    long? ....
    ....

    ....
    ....

13. Are you a smoker and for how long?..
    ....

14. Do you work as a chimney sweep and for how long? ....

15. Do you heat with a stove using wood, coal, oil, pellets, or biomass? If so, for
    how long (at home and at work)? ....
    ....

    ....
    ....

16. Are you exposed to tobacco smoke at home or at work and for how long (during the day and in total)? ....
....
....
....

17. Where do you live and work: in an urban, rural, or semi-urban environment? For how long? .....
....
....
....
....

18. Are you exposed to exhaust gases from motor vehicles or trains? If so, how many days and for how long? ....
....
....

19. Have you recently (when and how much) consumed charred food?...................
....
....
....

20. Are you a griller or do you often grill food (how often)?...........................
....
....

21. Do you work as a firefighter? If you work, when was the last time you were exposed to fire or smoke and for how long? ....
....
....
....

22. Have you recently been exposed to a fire (forest fire, city fire)? If so, when and for how long? ....
....
....

23. Have you consumed grilled, smoked, or fried food in the last 2 days? If so, when and how much? ....
....
....

24. Do you work or live near the industry: cement, bitumen, car tires, asphalt, petrochemical, or coke? If you work, how long have you been working and what jobs? If you live near the mentioned industries, how long have you lived there and at what distance from them?..
....
....
....
....
....

25. Do you consume food produced within a radius of 15 km from the mentioned industries? If so, when was the last time you consumed it, which food, and in what quantity? ....

....

....

....

....

26. Do you work as a car mechanic? If so, when and for how long?

....

....

27. Do you work with lubricants or as a professional driver? If so, when and for how long?...

....

....

....

28. Do you work in the railways? If so, in what jobs and for how long? .....

....

....

Chapter 26

1. Do you work in a place where you are exposed to smoke? If you work, for how long and in what jobs?...

....

....

....

2. Do you work in factories with blast furnaces, oxygen furnaces, or electric arc furnaces? If so, when and for how long?...

....

....

....

....

3. Do you work or live near an iron and steel foundry? If you work, how long have you been working and what jobs? If you live near an iron and steel foundry, how long have you lived there and how far from the foundry? ....

....

....

....

....

....

Chapter 27

1. Do you work with tar? If you work, for how long and in what jobs?
   ....
   ....

2. Do you work or live near the tar or tar resin industry and for how long? ....
   ....
   ....
   ....

3. Do you work in the parking lot, in what jobs, and for how long?.......................
   ....
   ....
   ....

4. Do you work or live near the bitumen industry and for how long?
   ....
   ....

5. Do you work as a street vendor? If so, when and for how long?.........................
   ....
   ....
   ....

6. Do you work in road companies, paving streets and roads, and making side-
   walks, in which jobs, and for how long? ....
   ....
   ....

7. Do you work or live near the tar industry, how far, and for how long? ....
   ....

Chapter 28

1. Did you work in coal mining and/or processing? If so, what jobs did you work
   and for how long? ....
   ....
   ....
   ....

2. Did you live near a place where coal was mined? If so, how long did you live
   near such a place and how far was the place where you lived from the place
   where the coal was mined? ....
   ....
   ....
   ....
   ....
   ....

3. Did you work on the purification of waste water from the coal industry? If so, what jobs did you work for and for how long? ....
   ....
   ....

4. Have you consumed food produced in the territory where coal was once extracted and/or processed (specify when)? If so, how long have you consumed it and which foods?
   ....
   ....
   ....
   ....
   ....
   ....

5. Have you worked on the removal of tailings from the coal industry? If so, what jobs did you work for and for how long? ....
   ....
   ....
   ....
   ....

6. Did you live near a place where tailings from the coal industry were disposed of? If so, how long have you lived near such a place and how far was the place where you lived from the place where the tailings from the coal industry were disposed of? ....
   ....
   ....
   ....
   ....

7. Have you consumed food produced in the territory where tailings from the coal industry (mine) were once (specify when) disposed of? If so, how long have you consumed it and which food?...
   ....
   ....
   ....
   ....
   ....

8. Do you work in the production of carbon electrodes, asbestos, or products containing asbestos? If so, in which jobs and for how long? ....
   ....
   ....
   ....

9. Do you work or live near an aluminum mine or industry and for how long? .....
   ....
   ....
   ....
   ....

10. Do you work or live near the refinery and for how long? ....
....
....

11. Do you work or live near the metal industry, chemical industry, or electrical industry and for how long? ....
....
....
....

12. Do you work or live near the mineral oil industry, how far, and for how long? ...
....
....

13. Do you work in the wood industry, in what jobs, and for how long? ....
....
....

Chapter 29

1. Do you work with municipal waste, hospital waste, hazardous waste, and sewage sludge? If so, in which jobs and for how long? ....
....
....
....

2. Do you work in the cement industry, or with cement? If so, in what jobs and for how long? ....
....
....
....

3. Do you work or live near the pulp and paper industry, chemical industry (chemical production of chlorophenol, vinyl chloride; pulp bleaching, production of phenoxy herbicides), or metal industry (smelting and refining of metals)? What jobs have you been working on and for how long? How far do you live from the mentioned industries?
....
....
....
....

4. Do you work or live near a coal plant? What jobs have you been working on and for how long? How far do you live from the mentioned facilities? ....
....
....
....

5. Do you use diesel vehicles or are you exposed to exhaust gases from diesel vehicles? If so, for how long and in what situations? ....
....
....
....
....

6. Do you work or live near a crematorium? What jobs have you been working on and for how long? How far do you live from the mentioned facilities? ....
....
....
....

7. Do you work or live near an incinerator? What jobs have you been working on and for how long? How far and how long have you lived from the mentioned facilities? ....
....
....
....

8. In the last 3 days, have you been exposed to forest or similar fires, wood burning, photolytic, or biochemical processes accompanied by the release of gases? If so, by what processes, for how long, and in what capacity? ....
....
....
....
....
....

9. Have you consumed egg yolks, fatty dairy products, or fish in the last 3 days? If so, in what quantities, which dairy products, and which fish? Does the fish belong to the salmonids and was it caught in estuaries? ....
....
....
....
....
....

10. Have you consumed a large amount of meat in the last 3 days? If yes, in what quantities and which meat?..
....
....
....

11. Have you consumed caviar or fish roe in the last 2 days? If so, in what quantities and where do the mentioned products come from?..
....
....
....

12. Have you consumed shellfish or fatty food in the last 2 days? If so, in what quantities and where do the mentioned products come from?...................................
....
....
....

13. Do you consume food produced at the sites of former incinerators, landfills, or river sediments? ....
....
....
....
....
....

14. Do you work or live near a secondary copper smelter? What jobs have you been working on and for how long? How far and how long have you lived from the mentioned facilities? ....
....
....
....

15. Do you reside or live near major roads, intersections, freight routes, or bus stations? How far and how long have you lived from the mentioned facilities?
....
....
....
....

16. Do you work or live near a coal-fired thermal power plant? What jobs have you been working on and for how long? How far and how long have you lived from the mentioned facilities? ....
....
....
....
....

17. Do you work or live near industrial boilers? What jobs have you been working on and for how long? How far and how long have you lived from the mentioned facilities? ....
....
....
....

18. Do you work or live near an iron ore sintering plant? What jobs have you been working on and for how long? How far and how long do you live from the mentioned facilities? ....
....
....
....

19. Have you stayed in the territory of Vietnam or consumed food originating from the territory of Vietnam where "Agent Orange" was used during the American-Vietnam War?
    If you did stay in the incriminated areas, when and how long did you stay there and in what capacity? ....
    ....
    ....
    ....
    If you consumed food originating from the territory of Vietnam where "Agent Orange" was used during the US-Vietnam War, when did you consume it, what type of food, and how much? ....
    ....
    ....
    ....

20. Do you work or live near a tannery, varnish, pigment, or paint factory? What jobs have you been working on and for how long? How far away and how long have you lived near the mentioned facilities? ....
    ....
    ....
    ....
    ....
    ....

21. Do you work or live near a landfill, plastic factory, or electric transformer cooling fluid (polychlorinated biphenyls) factory? What jobs have you been working on and for how long? How far away and how long have you lived near the mentioned facilities? ....
    ....
    ....
    ....

22. Have you breathed air filled with ash in the last 3 days? If so, when and for how long? Do you know the origin of ash?..
    ....
    ....
    ....
    ....
    ....

23. Do you work or live near a metal recycling center? What jobs have you been working on and for how long? How far away and how long have you lived near the mentioned facilities? ....
    ....
    ....
    ....
    ....
    ....

24. In the last 2 days, have you been intensively exposed to exhaust gases from motor vehicles or exhaust gases from organic fuel heaters? If so, when and for how long? Do you know the origin of heating element fuel? ....
....
....

25. Do you work or live near the fungicide or herbicide industry? What jobs have you been working on and for how long? How far away and how long have you lived near the mentioned facilities? ....
....
....
....
....
....

26. In the last 2 days, have you consumed food or drink (wine) from the territory where fungicides and/or herbicides were intensively applied? If so, in what quantities and where do the mentioned products come from?..........................
....
....
....

27. In the last 2 days, have you been exposed to facilities where chlorine is used? If so, when and for how long? Do you know what kind of plants, processes, or products these are?...
....
....
....
....
....

28. Have you been exposed to (worked with) the contents of electrical transformers or capacitors in the last few days? If so, when and for how long? What exactly did you do on the said devices? ....
....
....
....
....
....

29. Do you work or live near a steel mill, bar smelter, or electric arc furnace plant? What jobs have you been working on and for how long? How far and for how long have you lived near the mentioned facilities? ....
....
....
....
....
....

Chapter 30

1. Do you work in a carpet cleaning service? What jobs have you been working on and for how long? How far away and how long have you lived near the mentioned service? ....
....
....
....
....

2. Do you work in the industry of refrigerants (appliances or chemicals)? What jobs have you been working on and for how long? How far and how long have you lived near the listed industry? Do you consume food produced or water originating from the territory where the mentioned industry was or is loca ted?..
....
....
....
....

3. Do you work in the degreasing, thinner or degreasing solvent industry? What jobs have you been working on and for how long? How far and how long have you lived near the listed industry? Do you consume food produced or water originating from the territory where the mentioned industry was or is loca ted?..
....
....
....
....

4. Do you work in the chemical paint and varnish remover industry or in the adhesive industry? What jobs have you been working on and for how long? How far and how long have you lived near the listed industry? Do you consume food produced or water originating from the territory where the mentioned industry was or is located?
....
....
....
....

5. Do you work in the chemical metal tool cleaner, cleaning wipes or chemical stain remover industry? What jobs have you been working on and for how long? How far and how long have you lived near the listed industry? Do you consume food produced or water originating from the territory where the mentioned industry was or is located? ....
....
....
....
....
....

6. Do you work in a dry cleaning service? What jobs have you been working on and for how long? How far away and how long have you lived near the mentioned service?...............................

....

....

....

....

7. Did you work on oiling weapons, tools, or other equipment in the army? If so, what jobs exactly did you work for and how long? How far and how long have you lived near the activity? Do you consume food produced or water originating from the territory where the mentioned activity was or is being carried out?

....

....

....

....

....

8. Are there people suffering from kidney, liver, prostate, esophagus, or non-Hodgkin's lymphoma in your business or residence environment? If they exist, how long have they been working with you or living in your environment? ......

....

....

....

....

9. Do you work in the production of liquid for correction of written material, industries: wood finishing, cleaning agents, polishing agents, or lubricants? What jobs have you been working on and for how long? How far and how long have you lived near the listed industries? Do you consume food produced or water originating from the territory where the mentioned industries were or are located?...

....

....

....

....

10. Do you work in the textile dyeing, printing, or laundry/cleaning industries? What jobs have you been working on and for how long? How far and how long have you lived near the listed industries? Do you consume food produced or water originating from the territory where the mentioned industries/businesses were or are located?.......................

....

....

....

....

11. Do you work on cleaning/degreasing in the industry: electronics, microelectronics, telecommunications, optics, rubber and rubber products, mineral products, transport equipment, or metal products? What jobs have you been working on and for how long? How far and how long have you lived near the listed industries? Do you consume food produced or water originating from the territory where the mentioned industries/businesses were or are located? ....

12. Do you work in the aviation industry, the watch industry, or the weapons industry? What jobs have you been working on and for how long? How far and how long have you lived near the listed industries? Do you consume food produced or water originating from the territory where the mentioned industries/businesses were or are located?...............................

13. Do you work in the pesticide, distillery, marine equipment, oil refining, radar, or footwear industries? What jobs have you been working on and for how long? How far and how long have you lived near the listed industries? Do you consume food produced or water originating from the territory where the mentioned industries/businesses were or are located? ....

14. Do you work in embalming, with resins, construction or maintenance of sewage, silk industry, taxidermy of birds and animals, or maintenance of work systems? What jobs have you been working on and for how long? How far and how long have you lived near the listed industries? Do you consume food produced or water originating from the territory where the mentioned industries/businesses were or are located?

15. Do you work in waste or landfill work, or as a tobacco denicotinizer? What jobs exactly have you been working on and for how long? How far and how long have you lived near the listed industries? Do you consume food produced or water originating from the territory where the mentioned industries/businesses were or are located?.......

....

....

....

....

16. Do you live in a place where there used to be a military base, military warehouses, or any of the listed incriminated industries/businesses? If you live in such a place, which of the incriminated activities were carried out there, for how long, and how much time has passed since then? ....

....

....

....

17. Are there children in your area with rhabdomyosarcomas (malignant diseases of the soft tissues of children) or children with brain tumors? If so, do they live near the incriminated industries (places) and for how long? Did their mothers live in such places during pregnancy? ....

....

....

....

....

....

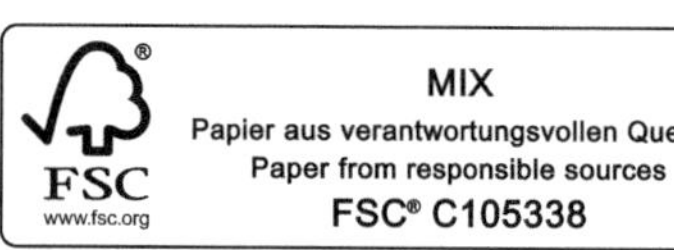

If you have any concerns about our products,
you can contact us on
ProductSafety@springernature.com

In case Publisher is established outside the EU,
the EU authorized representative is:
**Springer Nature Customer Service Center GmbH
Europaplatz 3, 69115 Heidelberg, Germany**

Printed by Libri Plureos GmbH
in Hamburg, Germany